Principles of Dentoalveolar Extractions

Principles of Dentoalveolar Extractions

Seth Delpachitra
Anton Sklavos
Ricky Kumar

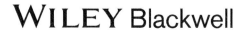

Registered Offices
John Wiley & Sons, Inc., 111 River Street, Hoboken, NJ 07030, USA
John Wiley & Sons Ltd, The Atrium, Southern Gate, Chichester, West Sussex, PO19 8SQ, UK

Editorial Office
9600 Garsington Road, Oxford, OX4 2DQ, UK

For details of our global editorial offices, customer services, and more information about Wiley products visit us at www.wiley.com.

Wiley also publishes its books in a variety of electronic formats and by print-on-demand. Some content that appears in standard print versions of this book may not be available in other formats.

Library of Congress Cataloging-in-Publication Data
Names: Delpachitra, Seth Navinda, 1988– author. | Sklavos, Anton William,
  1990- author. | Kumar, Ricky Ritesh, 1976– author.
Title: Principles of dentoalveolar extractions / Seth Navinda Delpachitra,
  Anton William Sklavos, Ricky Ritesh Kumar.
Description: Hoboken, NJ : Wiley-Blackwell, 2020. | Includes
  bibliographical references and index.
Identifiers: LCCN 2020025027 (print) | LCCN 2020025028 (ebook) | ISBN
  9781119596400 (cloth) | ISBN 9781119596417 (adobe pdf) | ISBN
  9781119596448 (epub)
Subjects: MESH: Tooth Extraction–methods
Classification: LCC RK531 (print) | LCC RK531 (ebook) | NLM WU 605 | DDC
  617.6/6–dc23
LC record available at https://lccn.loc.gov/2020025027
LC ebook record available at https://lccn.loc.gov/2020025028

Cover Design: Wiley
Cover Image: Seth Delpachitra

Set in 9.5/12.5pt STIXTwoText by SPi Global, Pondicherry, India

SKYD3050B69-4861-452A-9790-6107AA954A1B_011221

Contents

Foreword

The attachment of teeth to bone, facilitated by the periodontal ligament, is a unique connective tissue articulation. It enables tooth eruption, appropriate physiological responses to compressive force, and planned orthodontic tooth movement. However, as odontogenic infections may be potentially fatal, specialised skills for efficient tooth extraction have evolved from the days of the 'barber-surgeons' of the Middle Ages to contemporary exodontia. Today, every conceivable type of useful instrumentation and imaging is available to the clinician.

Tooth removal in the middle of the last century occupied a large part of the dental practitioner's work and skill set, but this has markedly reduced due to better dental care and tooth maintenance. The time devoted to the discipline of exodontia in the dental curriculum has thus diminished proportionally, and many graduates emerge with minimal experience in removing teeth. A fresh, comprehensive guide to the principles of dentoalveolar extractions for all interested practitioners who wish to underpin their clinical experience with clear guidelines is therefore most welcome.

In a logical sequence, the authors have addressed all aspects of managing a patient for simple and surgical extractions. By introducing the 'principles of surgery' from the outset, the reader is reminded that tooth removal is within the surgical spectrum and carries the same responsibilities in terms of providing careful patient assessment, consent, a controlled clinical environment, and necessary documentation. A detailed knowledge of the associated anatomy and competence in the administration of local anaesthesia are fundamental for successful dentoalveolar surgery in the outpatient setting and are well covered in this book, as are the available surgical instruments.

A methodical approach in performing simple and surgical extractions, including the management of intraoperative events and third molar surgery, is also provided, with headings for assessment, equipment, and patient position. These chapters are supported by good-quality anatomical diagrams to assist in the understanding of the suggested techniques.

With our ageing population, there are many medications and diseases that must be thoroughly understood by the dental practitioner. A chapter on medical compromise is an important addition to this text as it covers issues such as the newer anticoagulant agents and medications for bone loss that influence healing. The taking of these drugs may significantly modify a treatment plan, and decisions regarding joint management with the patient's prescribing physician are often indicated. Finally, postoperative care and complications are discussed, as these represent vital knowledge in surgical care.

Many books covering this field have included chapters devoted to exodontia, as part of a broader spectrum of oral and maxillofacial surgery. However, this neat, clear, and inclusive volume fulfills the objective of providing a modern reference text devoted to dentoalveolar surgery alone. It will instruct all those who set out to master the skills of exodontia in their practising lives, from under-graduate students to surgical trainees and newly qualified dental practitioners. I have no doubt that this excellent resource will be consumed and enjoyed by many in the years to come.

Professor Andrew A.C. Heggie, AM
Oral and Maxillofacial Surgeon
Melbourne, Australia

About the Companion Website

Don't forget to visit the companion website for this book:

www.wiley.com/go/delpachitradentoalveolarextractions

There you will find valuable material designed to enhance your learning, including:

- MCQs

Scan this QR code to visit the companion website.

1

Principles of Surgery

> **surgery** *n. manual treatment of injuries or disorders of the body, operative therapeutics.*
> **surgeon** *n. a person skilled in surgery.*

Exodontia, the removal of teeth, involves the manipulation of hard and soft tissues and the amputation of the dentition or parts thereof in order to treat or prevent disease, or as part of an overall treatment plan. The surgeon who carries out this treatment must possess qualities, skills, and decision-making abilities to the standard of any other trained surgeon who diagnoses and treats disease. It is the responsibility of this surgeon to provide the highest standard of care of which they are capable, and when they cannot provide it to a suitable level, to refer to the appropriate specialist service.

It is somewhat self-evident, though easily forgotten, that the surgeon's responsibility is not limited to the operation only, but also involves preoperative consultation and postoperative monitoring, as well as other aspects of care such as liaising with other practitioners and communicating treatment plans. Surgeons are trained to possess several qualities and characteristics not limited to procedural skills:

- **Knowledge.** Knowledge can be considered the facts, information, skills, and experience gained through education, training, and professional practice. It is a fundamental and essential aspect of the carrying out of dentoalveolar extractions. It includes technical and medical expertise, which facilitate safe patient management. As scientific knowledge evolves over time, there is a need for ongoing maintenance through continuing professional development and keeping up to date with evidence-based practice.
- **Quality and Safety.** Quality is the commitment to excellence, providing a service that is guided primarily by the best interests of the patient. This is achieved through recognition of one's own strengths and limitations, stringent self-audit, and the fortitude to request assistance when needed. Safety is the avoidance of risk or injury to oneself, one's staff, and one's patients. Maintenance of a safe workplace is the responsibility of all individuals employed in a health environment, and requires appropriate training and awareness of risk-mitigation strategies such as aseptic and sterilisation techniques. Quality and safety are dynamic components of surgery and necessitate constant refinement and improvement to ensure the wellbeing of patients and a high standard of care.
- **Communication and Collaboration.** Good communication is essential in the interaction both with patients and with other health professionals. Clear, concise, and relevant documentation of patient management will improve interactions with specialists and foster a culture of collaboration and professional development. This is particularly important when patients are

undergoing tooth extraction as part of a wider treatment plan where multiple other medical comorbidities require interdisciplinary management. In such situations, good communication minimises delays to receiving time-critical treatment, such as in the case of dental extractions prior to head and neck radiotherapy or bisphosphonate treatment.

- **An Individualistic Approach.** Patients will have a wide variety of backgrounds, demands, and prior medical knowledge. A tailored and individualised approach is required in order to ensure they understand the proposed procedure, its risks, and its expected outcomes, and are able to compare options in order to make an informed decision.
- **Leadership and Management.** A surgeon will often find themselves the leader of a multifaceted treatment team, including nursing staff, dental assistants, anaesthetic staff, and sterilisation technicians. This leadership comes with great responsibility: the expert surgeon must guide others in the team, provide feedback and education, and thus help maintain a standard of excellence. The surgeon must ensure that all staff are orientated towards the goal of achieving the best outcome for the patient. When the highest standard of care is compromised, the responsibility is on the surgeon to make sure the team gets back on track.
- **Decision Making.** The word 'decision' shares a common root with another word often associated with surgery: incision. Both are derivatives from the Latin word *caedis*, meaning 'to cut'. Incision means to cut into something, such as the operative site; decision literally means 'to cut away'. A decision thus precludes other options, and sets one upon a particular course of action. A skilled surgeon will be able to make treatment planning decisions that are in the best interests of their patients.

1.1 Wound Healing

Good outcomes following surgery depend on satisfactory wound healing. This involves a range of inflammatory, biochemical, and physiologic changes at the operative site, which will ultimately lead to resolution, healing, and bone remodelling. Wound healing does not always follow a predictable course, and therefore an understanding of its key aspects will serve as a foundation for interpreting clinical signs and determining when it is compromised.

There are four key stages in wound healing (Figure 1.1):

1) Haemostasis.
2) Inflammatory phase.
3) Proliferative phase.
4) Remodelling and resolution.

An interruption at any one of these stages will lead to a protracted recovery period.

1.1.1 Haemostasis

Any tissue trauma will result in bleeding from the local vasculature supplying the tissues. The immediate physiologic reaction is haemostasis, which involves reactive vasospasm, formation of a platelet plug, and activation of the coagulation cascade.

Reactive vasospasm occurs in the seconds to minutes following damage to the blood vessels. This is mediated through neurologic mechanisms, as well as the local release of endothelin. It rapidly reduces blood loss from trauma. In surgery, exogenous vasoactive medications such as adrenaline utilise this response to improve visual access to the surgical field by reducing blood flow.

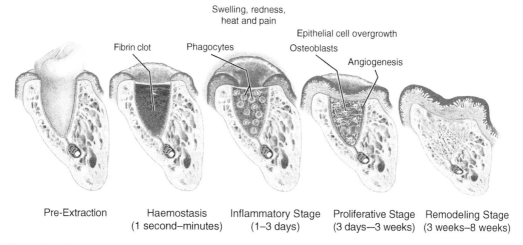

Figure 1.1   Phases of wound healing.

Damaged endothelial cells result in a conformational change in von Willebrand factor expressed on the cell surface. Von Willebrand factor interacts with glycoprotein Ib on circulating platelets, resulting in activation and aggregation of the platelets, forming links to fibrinogen via the GpIIb/IIIa receptor. This leads to the formation of the platelet plug. Antiplatelet medications inhibit aspects of platelet plug formation and increase the risk of bleeding during surgical procedures.

The coagulation cascade is a series of successive reactions that occur in order to activate thrombin and form a stable fibrin clot (Figure 1.2). There are two pathways in this cascade: intrinsic and extrinsic. The intrinsic pathway is activated within the vascular system through exposure

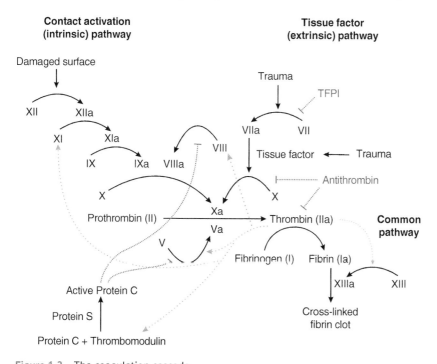

Figure 1.2   The coagulation cascade.

to endothelial collagen, whilst the extrinsic pathway is activated by tissue trauma and release of intracellular tissue factor. Anticoagulant medications and coagulopathies increase the tendency to bleed by inhibiting aspects of the coagulation cascade, and awareness of these effects may be clinically relevant in surgical planning.

Coagulation studies used clinically can assess the function of either the intrinsic, the extrinsic, or the shared common pathway. Prothrombin time screens for factors II, V, VII, and X and fibrinogen; these are all part of the extrinsic pathway, which is used to guide treatment for patients treated with warfarin. Warfarin inhibits vitamin K-dependent factors common to both pathways, but because factor VII has the shortest half-life, the extrinsic pathway is used to determine coagulability. The partial thromboplastin time will screen for factors in the intrinsic pathway affected by medications such as heparin and low-molecular-weight heparin.

1.1.2   Inflammatory Phase

This will commence on day one after the procedure and will continue for approximately three days. Important aspects of the inflammatory response include the release of pro-inflammatory mediators and vasoactive factors such as the prostaglandins, leukotrienes, interleukins, and histamine, and recruitment of phagocytes to remove dead tissue and foreign debris. The inflammatory mediators lead to the swelling, redness, heat, pain, and loss of function associated with inflammation. Anti-inflammatory medications are commonly prescribed after dentoalveolar procedures in order to mitigate the postoperative pain and swelling.

1.1.3   Proliferative Phase

This typically starts around day three and lasts for up to three weeks. The proliferative phase relies on the formation of granulation tissue and type III collagen, mediated by fibroblasts; wound contraction starts due to the action of myofibroblasts. Angiogenesis takes place as new capillaries are formed to provide blood and nutrients in order to help the wound heal. A number of growth factors, including vascular endothelial growth factor (VEGF), are also involved. At the wound edges, epithelial cells proliferate and begin to grow over the granulation tissue scaffold that has formed. Bone healing starts to take place as osteoprogenitor cells arrive, differentiating into osteoblasts, which begin depositing an osteoid matrix. Note that any systemic conditions or medications which prevent or suppress components of angiogenesis or inflammation may delay or prolong healing.

1.1.4   Remodelling and Resolution

At the completion of three weeks of healing, granulation tissue and immature bone will fill the extraction site, and the socket should be completely covered by a layer of epithelium. Bone remodelling will continue to take place with active resorption and deposition mediated by osteoblasts and osteoclasts. This important step can be impeded by medications that inhibit osteoclast function, such as bisphosphonates or denosumab. Radiographic evidence of bone remodelling will not become evident until after six to eight weeks.

1.2   Patient Assessment

Any medical or dental intervention requires a comprehensive patient history. This includes: a detailed medical history, including current and past medical treatments; documentation of known drug allergies and reactions; a social history comprising occupation and use of alcohol, cigarettes, and illicit substances; prior surgeries, dental treatments, and adverse outcomes; and, finally, the patient's chief complaint or main concerns.

Secondary to this is the clinical assessment of the patient's orofacial region, including both extraoral and intraoral examination. This should include an assessment of the temporomandibular joint, soft and hard tissue pathologies, and the presence of any dental pathology. Simultaneously, a difficulty and risk assessment for dentoalveolar surgery can be undertaken, paying particular attention to mouth opening, gingival biotype, gag reflex, patient anxiety, and previous heavily restored dentition.

Diagnostic tests should be carried out as necessary, including pulp testing, palpation for mobility, and percussion testing. A periodontal probe can be used to examine partially erupted or unerupted teeth, to assess soft tissue opercula, or to explore other communications with the oral cavity.

The patient's psychological state and level of anxiety can be assessed by asking how well they have tolerated dental treatment in the past. This aspect of the assessment is important; by virtue of temperament, some patients will require a more detailed discussion about their treatment, and some may request or require treatment with sedation or general anaesthesia.

1.3 Radiographic Assessment

Plain-film orthopantomogram (OPG), periapical (PA) radiograph, and the three-dimensional (3D) cone-beam computed tomogram (CBCT) are the primary imaging modalities used in the assessment of patients prior to dental extractions. As part of the radiographic workup for dental extraction, the minimum required imaging of the tooth for extraction is an intraoral PA radiograph. Where multiple teeth are indicated for extraction, or where third molars are being assessed, a panoramic radiograph is the minimum requirement instead (Figure 1.3).

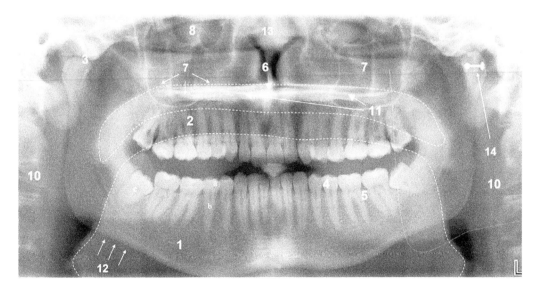

Figure 1.3   Panoramic radiograph: 1. mandible; 2. maxilla; 3. temporomandibular joint; 4. dentition; 5. alveolar process and periodontium; 6. anterior nasal spine; 7. maxillary antrum; 8. orbit; 9. zygoma; 10. cervical spine (double image); 11. hard palate (double image); 12. lower border of mandible; 13. nasal septum; 14. earring causing artifact. Outlines show oro- and nasopharyngeal airspaces and double image of mandibular ramus (left side). *Source:* Reproduced from The panoramic dental radiograph for emergency physicians by Anton Sklavos, Daniel Beteramia, Seth Navinda Delpachitra, Ricky Kumar, *BMJ* 36: 565–571. doi:10.1136/emermed-2018-208332. Copyright © 2019 with permission from BMJ Publishing Group Ltd.

A procedure should not be undertaken without a diagnostic radiograph, displaying the condition of the tooth, the relevant adjacent structures (inferior alveolar nerve canal, mental foramen, maxillary antrum), and the condition of the adjacent teeth. Generally, a PA radiograph has a limited application and should only be used for emergency single-tooth extractions or procedures limited to one part of the mouth performed under local anaesthesia. A PA radiograph is not considered an appropriate assessment for proximity of the inferior alveolar canal to the lower third molar teeth; errors in patient or film positioning may alter the radiographic relationship between the canal and associated tooth roots, producing a nondiagnostic image.

The OPG gives a better indication of the overall state of the patient's dentition and of other pathological conditions that may affect the maxillofacial region compared to a PA radiograph. Because the OPG is taken in a standardised manner, it has formed the basis for a number of evidence-based risk-assessment tools in the current literature, including assessments of the risk of oroantral communication and inferior alveolar nerve injury.

CBCT is a relatively new and inexpensive method of producing 3D images of maxillomandibular structures (Figure 1.4). It is indicated when conventional 2D imaging does not produce enough diagnostic information for treatment planning. Most commonly, this is to investigate jaw

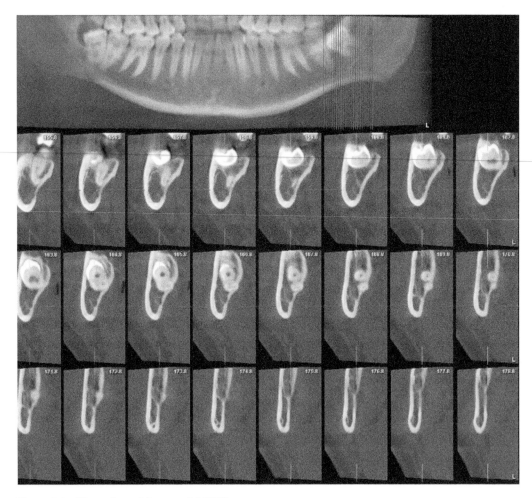

Figure 1.4 Slices of a serial transaxial CBCT.

pathology or the relationship of the inferior alveolar nerve canal to third molar teeth. Whilst CBCT images come in a variety of formats, the serial-transaxial reformat is useful for the determination of the pathway of the inferior alveolar nerve and its relationship to the mandibular teeth.

CBCT images provide a great deal more information than plain-film imaging, and therefore their interpretation can be challenging. For the surgeon who is not experienced with CBCT images, formal reporting by a specialist radiologist is essential; if they are not interpreted carefully, radiographic signs of nerve risk or bone pathology may be easily missed, likely resulting in a poor outcome for the patient and a litigious scenario for the surgeon.

1.4 Informed Consent

In order to carry out any medical or dental procedure, consent must be obtained from either the patient or their legal guardian. A valid consent may only be given when the patient possesses decision-making capacity; that is, when they have the ability to weigh up the pros and cons of treatment and come to a sound decision to either undergo or forgo a proposed procedure. This consent must be given voluntarily, without duress or coercion. The decision must be informed, which is to say that the patient must understand the procedure, the expected outcomes, the risks involved, the anticipated recovery time, and the costs of treatment.

For any planned surgical procedure, consent should be both written and verbal, and patients should be provided by the surgeon with a formal document detailing the procedure and its indications, risks, and expected outcomes (Figure 1.5). When seeking consent from a patient, the surgeon must always provide them sufficient time to ask questions. The patient may request more detailed information about particular risks or outcomes of surgery, and these should be elaborated on and explained in detail.

In addition, the consent should be specific for the particular patient and their individual circumstances. Alternatives to dentoalveolar extraction should be explained, and the reasons for and against their adoption detailed. In cases where extractions will render the patient without functional teeth, future treatment options for replacement should be discussed; this should include an approximate timeline, who will provide the treatment, and a rough cost estimate.

1.5 Anaesthesia

There are a number of different methods of anaesthesia available for dentoalveolar extractions. These include:

- Local anaesthesia only.
- Local anaesthesia with relative analgesia.
- Local anaesthesia with minor oral sedation.
- Local anaesthesia with intravenous (IV) sedation.
- Local anaesthesia with general anaesthesia.

Local anaesthesia alone can be administered for in-chair treatment, and is generally considered the safest option. It is appropriate for most simple dentoalveolar procedures and extractions. The main limitation of local anaesthesia is that it may be unsuitable for complex procedures, when a duration of more than 40 minutes is anticipated, or when the patient is anxious or otherwise uncooperative.

CONSENT FOR ORAL & MAXILLOFACIAL SURGERY	UR NUMBER:
	SURNAME:
	GIVEN NAME/S:
	DATE OF BIRTH:

The doctor/dentist has explained that I/the patient have/has the following condition:

_____

This condition requires the following procedure:

_____

There are risks associated with undertaking this procedure. These risks include (please tick):

Expected Complications:
☐ postoperative pain
☐ minor bleeding or bruising
☐ dry socket, causing severe pain or discomfort
☐ normal post-operative swelling of the face

Specific Risks not otherwise mentioned (please specify):

Uncommon Complications:
☐ temporary or permanent facial numbness due to damage to the nerves supplying the lower lip, chin, and lower teeth
☐ loss of taste due to damage to the nerve supplying the tongue
☐ bleeding which may be significant and require transfusion
☐ post-operative infection, which may either require antibiotics or further surgery
☐ damage to surrounding structures, including the lips, teeth, and tongue
☐ fragments of tooth or bone left in the gum or jaw
☐ fragments of upper teeth entering the sinuses, requiring further surgery for removal
☐ creation of a communication between the sinus and the mouth, requiring further surgery
☐ chronic pain or problems of the temporomandibular (jaw) joints
☐ jaw fracture

In consultation with my doctor/dentist, this procedure will be performed under:

☐	☐
LOCAL ANAESTHETIC	**GENERAL ANAESTHETIC**
I will be awake and will have injections to numb the area.	I will be asleep for this procedure.

Patient Statement

I understand my/the patient's medical condition and the proposed treatment.
I acknowledge the risks as documented above as well as those specific to my/the patient's individual situation.
I understand that anaesthetic is required for this procedure and the processes involved with my/the patient's choice of anaesthetic.
I understand that treatment is provided in a day surgery unit, and that transfer to another institution may be required if there are immediate complications of surgery.
I have the right to change my mind at any time regarding the procedure and choice of anaesthetic.
I have had all questions answered by the doctor/dentist and consent to the above procedure.

NAME OF PATIENT/PARENT/GUARDIAN: _____ RELATIONSHIP TO PATIENT: _____

SIGNATURE: _____ DATE: _____

Doctor/Dentist Statement	**Witness/Interpreter's Statement**
I have explained to the patient or guardian the content in this consent form and am comfortable that the person signing this form has capacity to do so.	I have provided an explanation to the patient of this consent form and any verbal information given to the patient.

NAME OF DOCTOR/DENTIST: _____ NAME OF INTERPRETER/WITNESS: _____

DESIGNATION: _____ LANGUAGE: _____

SIGNATURE: _____ DATE: _____ SIGNATURE: _____ DATE: _____

Figure 1.5 Example consent form for dentoalveolar surgery.

Table 1.1 Comparisons between commonly used oral benzodiazepine sedatives.

Drug name	Dose	Onset
Temazepam	10–20 mg	30–120 minutes
Diazepam	10–15 mg	30–90 minutes
Oxazepam	15–30 mg	2–3 hours

Relative analgesia involves the use of inhaled agents, such as nitrous oxide, to produce conscious sedation. It can be used as an adjunct with local anaesthesia, to improve patient comfort without significant airway risk. Nitrous oxide is usually administered through a nasal hood at concentrations of 50–70%. The advantage of this method is that it can be titrated and rapidly adjusted. However, there is a variable dose–response relationship between individuals, and patients may experience a number of unpleasant side effects if too high a dose is administered. Use of relative analgesia requires additional training, and it is recommended that at least two trained personnel are present in the clinic room when employing this technique.

Oral sedation, when employed effectively, can provide a greater level of sedation than nitrous oxide. Common drug classes used for oral sedation include benzodiazepine and barbiturate medications (Table 1.1). These drugs have a significant depressant effect on the central nervous system, and hence carry the serious risk of respiratory depression and loss of airway reflexes. Therefore, the use of oral sedation should only be considered when the surgeon and clinic personnel are sufficiently trained in anaesthesia, resuscitation, and airway management.

IV sedation typically involves more powerful sedative agents, such as midazolam, propofol, or fentanyl. It can only be administered in a setting which is fully prepared for airway management, such as a hospital theatre. As with all methods of anaesthesia where the airway is not secure, there is a risk that the patient will aspirate on any foreign object present in their mouth. This can be particularly dangerous when their reflexes are not protecting the airway. The administration of IV sedation may only be undertaken by a suitably qualified medical specialist or dental specialist with advanced training.

General anaesthesia will render the patient completely unconscious, and involves securing the airway using a laryngeal mask or endotracheal tube. It should be provided by a specialist anaesthetist or a suitably qualified medical professional. Dentoalveolar extractions carried out under general anaesthesia involve a shared airway, and communication with the anaesthetist throughout the procedure is essential.

1.6 Preparation of Equipment

Preparation for dentoalveolar extractions must follow the principles of asepsis, with strict maintenance of an aseptic operative field (Figure 1.6). The fundamental reason for this is to prevent transmission of microorganisms, which may cause surgical-site infections, transmit bloodborne diseases, and prolong postoperative healing. Inadequate or insufficient adherence to appropriate aseptic techniques or inadequate sterilisation of surgical instruments can result in harm to patients.

In hospital settings, sterilisation of instruments is usually performed through a hospital-wide central sterile services department. In the clinic setting, surgeons and their staff are responsible for the setup and proper maintenance of appropriate sterilisation facilities.

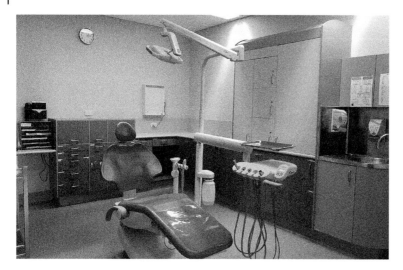

Figure 1.6   Clinic room with defined administrative, operative, and hygiene areas.

Prior to sterilisation, instruments should be wiped clear of obvious blood and debris, then cleaned in an ultrasonic (a machine that uses ultrasonic sound waves to vibrate instruments in order to remove small debris). The instruments should be wrapped or bagged, and chemical indicators that will change when sterilisation conditions are met placed on the equipment. Any practice that provides outpatient surgical procedures must ensure that staff are appropriately trained in sterilisation procedures and understand the basic minimum requirements.

Sterilisation of surgical equipment will fall into one of three categories: dry heat, moist heat, or sterilisation with gas. The sterilisation equipment must undergo regular and annual checks to ensure it is adequately maintained.

1.7   The Surgeon's Preoperative Checklist

When preparing for a procedure, the surgeon should run through a checklist to ensure that everything is in order. This includes:

- A signed consent (to be reviewed with the patient on the day of surgery).
- Confirmation of any allergies.
- A current radiograph, displayed in the surgical room (to be visible to the surgeon during the procedure).
- Confirmation of the correct side and site of the procedure.
- Use of personal protective equipment.
- Surgical handwash, gowning, and gloving.

The surgeon and trained staff should ensure that all equipment has been sterilised, is in suitable condition, and is handled in accordance with aseptic non-touch techniques. All equipment that is anticipated to be used or which may be required in the event of a complication should be ready. In some cases, it may be useful to have a 'scout' nurse to collect additional equipment as required.

Surgical Handrubbing Technique

- Handwash with soap and water on arrival to OR, after having donned theatre clothing (cap/hat/bonnet and mask).
- Use an alcohol-based handrub (ABHR) product for surgical hand preparation, by carefully following the technique illustrated in Images 1 to 17, before every surgical procedure.
- If any residual talc or biological fluids are present when gloves are removed following the operation, handwash with soap and water.

Put approximately 5ml (3 doses) of ABHR in the palm of your left hand, using the elbow of your other arm to operate the dispenser.

Dip the fingertips of your right hand in the handrub to decontaminate under the nails (5 seconds).

Images 3-7: Smear the handrub on the right forearm up to the elbow. Ensure that the whole skin area is covered by using circular movements around the forearm until the handrub has fully evaporated (10-15 seconds).

Images 8-10: Now repeat steps 1-7 for the left hand and forearm.

Put approximately 5ml (3 doses) of ABHR in the palm of your left hand as illustrated, to rub both hands at the same time up to the wrists, following all steps in images 12-17 (20-30 seconds).

Cover the whole surface of the hands up to the wrist with ABHR, rubbing palm against palm with a rotating movement.

Rub the back of the left hand, including the wrist, moving the right palm back and forth, and vice-versa.

Rub palm against palm back and forth with fingers interlinked.

Rub the back of the fingers by holding them in the palm of the other hand with a sideways back and forth movement.

Rub the thumb of the left hand by rotating it in the clasped palm of the right hand and vice versa.

When the hands are dry, sterile surgical clothing and gloves can be donned.

Repeat this sequence (average 60 sec) the number of times that adds up to the total duration recommended by the ABHR manufacturer's instructions. This could be two or even three times.

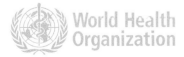
World Health Organization

Figure 1.7 WHO surgical handrubbing technique. *Source:* From Surgical Handrubbing Technique, https://www.who.int/gpsc/5may/hh-surgicalA3.pdf, WHO. © WHO.

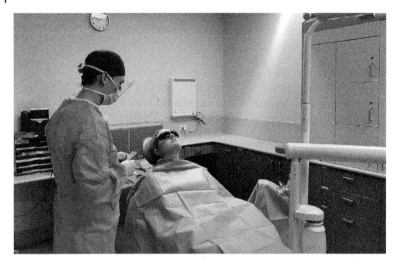

Figure 1.8 Dentist with sufficient sterile and personal protective attire for dentoalveolar surgery.

All surgical procedures require adequate lighting in order to visualise the operative field. This is particularly important when working in a small area such as the mouth. An overhead light should be used to ensure that both the surgeon and the assistant have adequate visual access to the field. The surgeon may also use a personal headlamp.

The surgeon should perform a surgical handwash prior to the procedure, as per the World Health Organization (WHO) surgical handrubbing technique, to ensure disinfection of contaminated skin of the hands, arms, and elbows (Figure 1.7). Typically, this will involve the use of a chlorhexidine- or iodine-based surgical handwash.

After the handwash, the surgeon must apply a sterile gown and gloves, so that they may enter the sterile field without contamination (Figure 1.8).

1.8 Operative Note

Following a surgical procedure, detailed clinical notes should be completed as soon as possible, listing all medications or anaesthetics administered and steps taken, the difficulty of the procedure, any intraoperative complications that arose, and any postoperative discussions with or instructions given to the patient. At a minimum, the operative note should include:

- Indications for the procedure and a summary of intraoperative findings.
- Type of anaesthesia used (relative anaesthesia, oral or IV sedation, general anaesthesia):
  - specifically, the type of local anaesthesia, dose administered, concentration, and use of vasoconstrictors.
- A detailed procedural note, including:
  - methods used for extraction ('simple' versus 'surgical'), with a detailed description of each step;
  - any complications encountered;
  - difficulty of the procedure;
  - haemostatic agents used;

- suture type;
- ease in obtaining haemostasis.
- Additional notes on any medications prescribed, including type, dose, and duration.
- Any postoperative orders that were given to the patient, and how they were transmitted (written, verbal, or both).
- The date and time of the follow-up appointment.

The operative note must reflect a legal memorandum outlining the specific intraoperative details of every case; a good clinical note enables continuity of care, provides a basis for informative evidence for any future complaints or complications, and enhances communication between healthcare professionals.

2

Local Anaesthesia

This chapter reviews the methods of obtaining sufficient local anaesthesia, an absolute necessity prior to performing any oral or dental surgery.

For most cases of dentoalveolar surgery, local anaesthesia alone – without any additional sedation – may provide sufficient patient comfort to allow the procedure to be completed. Local anaesthesia has an excellent safety profile, is readily accessible, and can be performed across a broad range of healthcare settings. Whilst other forms of anaesthesia can be powerful and effective, they entail multiple additional medical risks, necessitating additional training, equipment, and personnel prior to use. Ultimately, the decision over which method is most suitable will be made on the basis of informed consent and at the patient's discretion. However, the clinician should guide the patient through this decision based on their critical analysis of the expected outcomes, the ability of the patient to tolerate treatment, and a comprehensive review of the patient's medical history.

In certain scenarios, use of local anaesthesia alone may not be a suitable approach. Relative contraindications for performing awake dentoalveolar procedures include:

- Extraction of three or more teeth in a single procedure.
- A predicted high degree of intraoperative difficulty.
- An expected duration longer than 40 minutes.
- A high likelihood of major complications.
- Anxious or phobic patients.
- Extremes of patient age.
- The presence of associated pathology which may complicate the procedure.

Surgical procedures and dentoalveolar extractions in a dental clinic would be impossible without appropriate, safe, and effective local anaesthesia. This chapter outlines the fundamentals of local anaesthesia as it pertains to removal of teeth, including common preparations of anaesthetic agents, side effects, techniques, and troubleshooting when adequate anaesthesia is not achieved. Use of the local anaesthetic techniques outlined here requires an understanding of normal regional anatomy and innervation of the oral cavity.

Principles of Dentoalveolar Extractions, First Edition. Seth Delpachitra, Anton Sklavos and Ricky Kumar.
© 2021 John Wiley & Sons Ltd. Published 2021 by John Wiley & Sons Ltd.
Companion website: www.wiley.com/go/delpachitradentoalveolarextractions

2.1 Principles of Anaesthesia

1) **Patient Safety.** Patient safety is always the key priority in anaesthetic administration. This involves ensuring that the correct anaesthetic agent is utilised, there are no contraindications, the agent has not expired and has been stored correctly, and appropriate sterilisation and preparation have been carried out. Whenever injecting local anaesthesia, the clinician must ensure that they are up to date with cardiopulmonary resuscitation and are trained in the management of medical emergencies; local anaesthetic solutions may result in systemic side effects, and the patient should be monitored for such complications after administration.

2) **Informed Consent.** Local anaesthesia is not always well tolerated by patients, and this is largely due to patient expectations. For example, numbing of tongue sensation – a normal outcome of lingual nerve anaesthesia – may result in an anxious patient who feels unable to manage oral secretions. It is critical that patients are adequately informed of the expected effects of local anaesthesia; this is a key component of the informed consent process. The local and systemic risks must also be explained in detail as part of the overall procedural consent.

3) **Understanding of Regional Anatomy.** Effective local anaesthesia depends on delivery of a local anaesthetic agent to the appropriate nerves, tissues, or anatomic spaces. Similarly, avoidance of complications of local anaesthesia requires active avoidance of surrounding anatomic structures which may be encountered in similar anatomic areas. A sound knowledge of regional anatomy will ensure delivery of anaesthetic to the correct areas, whilst avoiding complications related to anatomic misadventure.

4) **Technical Expertise to Utilise Appropriate Techniques.** Surgeons who work in the oral cavity are technical experts in navigating the oral tissues, and the application of local anaesthesia is a skill that requires technical proficiency. The appropriate use of finger rests, retraction, and patient positioning can optimise patient comfort and tolerance of the procedure.

5) **Ability to Troubleshoot.** The surgeon performing anaesthesia must always think critically and determine potential reasons why local anaesthesia may have failed, including where additional techniques may be required to produce profound anaesthesia.

2.2 Mechanism of Action

Local anaesthetic agents produce their effect by reversibly blocking voltage-gated sodium ion channels in the axonal membranes of nerve cells, resulting in inhibition of action potential transmission along the axon (Figure 2.1). When local anaesthesia is applied to sensory nerves, painful stimuli are not conducted to the sensory cortex and pain is no longer perceived.

Local anaesthetic preparations are usually combined with a vasoconstrictive agent, commonly adrenaline or a synthetic vasopressin derivative (Figure 2.2). The concentration of local anaesthetic is typically given as a percentage, whilst the concentration of vasoconstrictor is given as a ratio (Table 2.1). The preparation may come in a dental cartridge, or in a vial to be drawn up before use. Before administering local anaesthetic, it is important to confirm the type, concentration, vasoconstrictor, and expiry date. Solutions with adrenaline have a number of advantages: the vasoconstrictive effect results in less haemorrhage in the operative field, allowing better visualisation; the duration of action is increased; and the risk of systemic toxicity is reduced. Whilst extremely rare, ischaemic cardiovascular complications may occur in patients with a prior history of cardiovascular disease, if preparations containing adrenaline are used in excess.

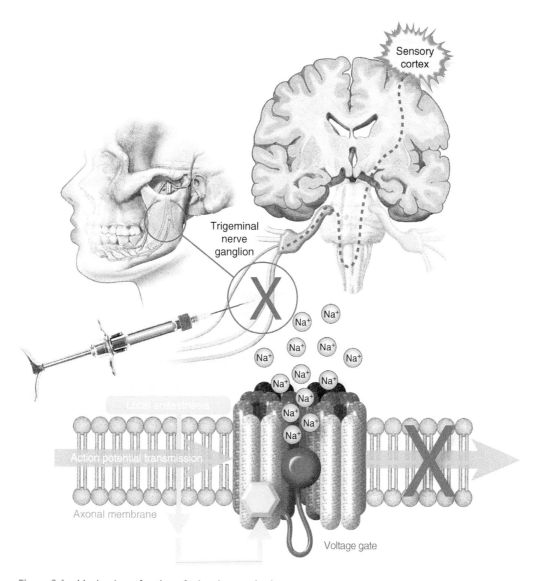

Figure 2.1   Mechanism of action of a local anaesthetic agent.

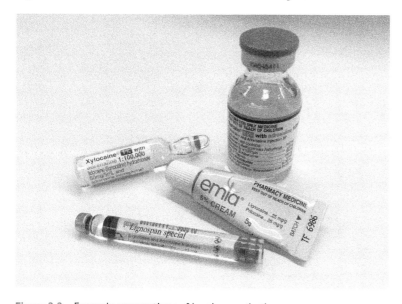

Figure 2.2   Example preparations of local anaesthetic.

Table 2.1 Conversion tables for local anaesthetic and adrenaline in solution.

Concentration	Dose
0.5% solution	5 mg/ml
1% solution	10 mg/ml
2% solution	20 mg/ml
4% solution	40 mg/ml
Concentration	Dose
1 : 80 000	12.5 µg/ml
1 : 100 000	10.0 µg/ml
1 : 200 000	5.0 µg/ml

2.3 Common Local Anaesthetic Preparations

Lignocaine is the most common agent used for local anaesthesia in dentistry. It is an amide-type anaesthetic with a rapid onset of action and an excellent safety profile, and when prepared with adrenaline, it has a duration of action of two to three hours, making it suitable for use in dentoalveolar extractions. It is commonly prepared as a 2% solution with 1 : 80 000 adrenaline. This provides 20 mg of lignocaine per millilitre of solution. The standard dental cartridge (2.2 ml) will deliver 44 mg of lignocaine. The maximum safe dose when prepared with adrenaline is 7 mg/kg.

Articaine has been in use for almost 20 years. It is advantageous for use in dental extractions due to its rapid onset of action and great diffusion potential. This is related to its unique molecular structure, which has both amide-like and ester-like bonds and an additional thiophene ring. These structures increase the lipid solubility of the molecule, whilst also making it susceptible to degradation by plasma esterases in the tissues. There is some controversy over its use in regional nerve blocks in dentistry, due to its association with increased neurotoxicity which may result in prolonged paraesthesia. Articaine is available in a 4% solution and is thought to provide a more profound anaesthesia than lignocaine when delivered as an infiltration. When prepared with adrenaline, the maximum dose is 7 mg/kg.

Bupivacaine is a local anaesthetic agent with a slower onset and longer duration of action than either lignocaine or articaine, with an anaesthetic effect of up to eight hours. Whilst this may be a disadvantage for procedures in the dental clinic setting, where rapid anaesthesia is desirable, it has the advantage of reducing the onset of postoperative discomfort. Bupivacaine is commonly prepared as a 0.5% solution with 1 : 200 000 adrenaline. The maximum safe dose is 2 mg/kg. Caution should be taken when administering bupivacaine because the dose leading to cardiotoxicity can precede symptoms associated with neurotoxicity. For most other anaesthetic agents, the reverse is true, and local anaesthetic overdose is more rapidly recognised.

Ropivacaine is a newer anaesthetic agent with similar characteristics to bupivacaine but a number of additional desirable qualities. It has a long duration of action of six hours and a comparably rapid onset. One unique benefit is that the molecule itself is vasoconstrictive, avoiding the need for additional vasoactive agents in its preparation. Additionally, there appears to be a lower risk of cardiotoxicity associated with the use of ropivacaine compared with bupivacaine. However, commercially available preparations are generally more expensive than other common anaesthetic agents used for dentoalveolar extractions.

2.4 Side Effects and Toxicity

In general, local anaesthetics are safe when used correctly. However, as with the administration of any pharmacological substance, there are risks that need to be considered and minimised.

2.4.1 Local Risks

A number of risks are inherently involved with the manipulation of deep-tissue planes and the injection of pharmacologically active substances into tissue spaces:

- Neuralgic-type pain from needle contact directly against a nerve trunk.
- Haematoma in the tissue space, resulting in trismus, pain, or visible bruising.
- Transient or permanent nerve injury from physical trauma or neurotoxicity of the anaesthetic agent.
- Needle breakage, leading to foreign-body complications.
- Transient facial paralysis due to the effect of anaesthetic on branches of the facial nerve.
- Necrotizing sialometaplasia, a rare ischaemic tissue reaction in response to trauma.

2.4.2 Systemic Risks

Systemic toxicity may occur after administration of local anaesthetic, particularly in paediatric or elderly populations. The risk is higher after inadvertent intravascular administration; a negative aspirate helps to reduce this risk. The initial signs are often related to the central nervous system, and include anxiety, dizziness, restlessness, tinnitus, and diplopia. If not recognised early, the patient may develop tremors, convulsions, and loss of consciousness. Late signs are related to cardiotoxicity, and include bradycardia, cardiovascular collapse, and cardiac arrest.

True allergic reactions to local anaesthetic are rare. Patients may report an 'allergy' after experiencing tachycardia or palpitations following administration of a local anaesthetic containing adrenaline, when in fact this is a normal physiologic response to the injection of vasoconstrictive medications. Patients may also be allergic to preservatives, or to latex in the bung of the cartridge. When a patient reports a previous adverse or allergic reaction, it is important to elicit the details to determine if it was a true allergy, which would involve rash, urticaria, oedema, and anaphylaxis. Ester local anaesthetic agents have a higher rate of allergic reaction than amide anaesthetic agents, attributed to a metabolite produced from degradation of the anaesthetic agent, p-aminobenzoic acid (PABA). Patients with sulphur allergies may experience a reaction to the metabisulphite additive used to stabilise adrenaline in solution.

2.5 Basic Oral Anaesthesia Techniques

Broadly, local anaesthetic techniques involving the oral cavity can be categorised into either infiltration-based techniques or regional nerve block techniques. Infiltration anaesthesia involves the injection of local anaesthetic agent directly adjacent to the surgical site, relying on diffusion of anaesthetic around small nerve branches and endings which supply the region to produce anaesthesia. Regional nerve block involves the injection of a local anaesthetic agent distant to the surgical site, around the known position of a larger nerve bundle that supplies the area. Regional nerve blocks can be used to anaesthetise the inferior alveolar nerve, including lingual branches, the long buccal nerve, the greater palatine, and nasopalatine nerves. Whilst a nerve block can be technically more challenging, as it relies on anatomic knowledge of nerve pathways in the head and neck, if performed correctly it can provide profound anaesthesia to larger anatomic areas with fewer injections, less local anaesthetic, and less patient discomfort.

2.5.1 Buccal Infiltration Anaesthetic

Buccal infiltration is a versatile technique that can be used to anaesthetise the maxillary dentition, the anterior mandible dentition, and the posterior mandible buccal mucosa (Figure 2.3). In anatomic areas where bone is thin and porous (e.g. anterior mandibular teeth or maxillary teeth), local anaesthetic solutions can diffuse through to the periodontium and tooth root apices, producing anaesthesia of the tooth itself. However, this technique does not adequately anaesthetise palatal or lingual tissues, which will need separate anaesthetic procedures prior to dental extraction. It likewise does not produce anaesthesia of the teeth or periodontal ligaments in the posterior mandible, due to the thick mandibular bony cortex; inferior alveolar nerve blocks will thus also be required.

1) Position the patient appropriately to ensure adequate access and lighting.
2) Retract the labial or buccal mucosa with a Minnesota retractor (or mouth mirror). Ensure adequate visualisation of attached and free gingiva. Keep the soft tissues taut to reduce patient discomfort.
3) Insert the needle into the deepest part of the vestibular sulcus in the buccal vestibule, and advance it approximately 2–3 mm, aiming for the approximate depth of the root apex but no further.
4) Aspirate the syringe to ensure the needle point has not traversed the intravascular space of a blood vessel.
5) Slowly inject the anaesthetic solution. A slow rate of injection will significantly reduce patient discomfort and pain.
6) Allow the local anaesthetic sufficient time to anaesthetise the tissues, based upon the pharmacokinetic properties of the anaesthetic solution, and monitor the patient for any adverse reaction.

Whilst infiltration anaesthesia is generally very safe, consideration should be given to regional structures. Insertion of the infiltration needle too deep into the maxillary vestibule can result in an unfortunate encounter with the orbit and its contents, whilst insertion too deep into the

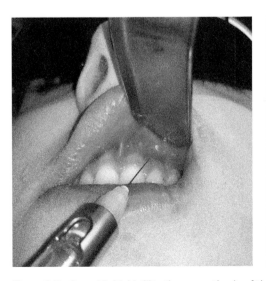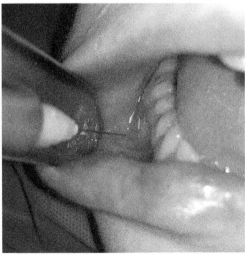

Figure 2.3   Buccal/labial infiltration anaesthesia of the maxilla (left) and mandible (right).

mandibular vestibule can lead to a puncture of the facial artery as it passes over the lower border of the mandible, resulting in a large haematoma.

2.5.2 Mandibular Teeth

Innervation to the mandibular teeth and their mucosa is supplied by the inferior alveolar nerve (including the mental and incisive branches), the lingual nerve, and the long buccal nerve. All are branches of the mandibular division of the trigeminal nerve, which travels inferiorly after exiting the cranium via the foramen ovale. On the medial aspect of the mandible at the level of the mandibular condyle, the main trunk branches; the buccal nerve travels anteriorly to innervate the buccal mucosa adjacent to the mandibular molars, whilst the inferior alveolar and lingual nerves travel inferiorly from the condyle on the medial aspect of the mandible, within the pterygomandibular space (Figure 2.4). The inferior alveolar nerve enters the mandible via the mandibular canal, and the lingual nerve, after its inferior descent, travels anteriorly to supply sensation to the lingual gingiva and anterior two-thirds of the tongue. The inferior alveolar nerve courses anteriorly within the mandible and exits via the mental foramen located on the outer cortex, near the apex of the mandibular first and second premolars. An incisive branch may continue within the mandible to supply the incisors.

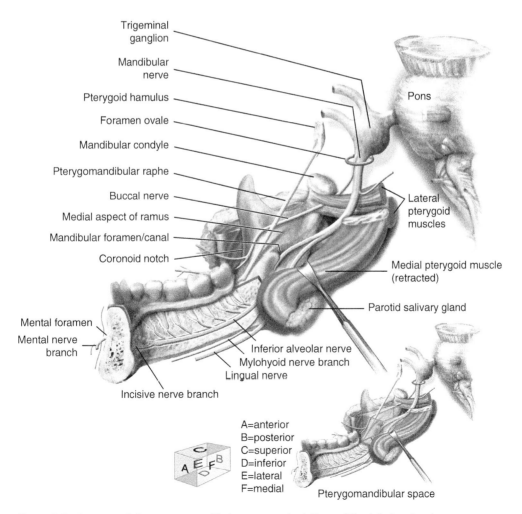

Figure 2.4 Anatomy of the pterygomandibular space and relations of the inferior alveolar nerve.

The critical anatomical space to visualise when performing any mandibular nerve block is the pterygomandibular space. This is formed by the medial aspect of the ramus (lateral), the medial pterygoid (medial), the pterygomandibular raphe (anterior), the parotid salivary gland (posterior), and superiorly by the lateral pterygoid. Several intraoral landmarks can be used together to identify the location of this space. The pterygotemporal depression can be identified between the raised edge of mucosa overlying the pterygomandibular raphe medially and that overlying the anterior border of the ramus laterally. The coronoid notch refers to the area of greatest convexity on the anterior border of the ramus; the inferior alveolar nerve and lingual nerve lie directly medial and posterior to it in the horizontal plane, approximately midway along the ramus. Within this space, the mandibular foramen lies approximately 1 cm above the occlusal plane of the lower molars; for any anaesthetic to be effective, injection into this space should ideally occur above this level. Injection too far posteriorly may result in inadvertent injection into the parotid gland where branches of the facial nerve lie, resulting in transient facial paralysis.

Injection of anaesthetic solution into the pterygomandibular space will affect both the inferior alveolar and lingual nerves, effectively anaesthetising the entire hemimandible, excluding the buccal mucosa and skin. Several techniques have been described for anaesthetising these two nerves; selection amongst them for an individual case depends on operator preference, clinical indication, and patient factors.

2.5.2.1 Conventional 'Open-Mouth' Technique

1) Position the patient in the dental chair, lying flat with head slightly extended and mouth open.
2) With the patient's mouth open, retract the buccal tissues to place tension on the pterygomandibular soft tissues and obtain sufficient vision and access. The pterygomandibular raphe can usually be visualised. Palpate the anterior border of the ramus to confirm the anatomic location of the pterygomandibular fold.
3) The site of needle penetration is approximately 1 cm above the occlusal plane of the mandibular teeth, into the pterygotemporal depression (Figure 2.5). The angle of insertion of the needle should be such that the barrel of the syringe is aligned with the contralateral premolar teeth. Advance the needle slowly through the soft tissues. As the needle is advanced, it will pierce through buccinator, through to the pterygomandibular space. If the orientation is correct, the needle will contact the medial aspect of the bony ramus near the mandibular canal after having advanced 2–2.5 cm.
4) Retract the needle 1–2 mm so that the needle point is within the pterygomandibular space. Confirm a negative aspirate using the syringe plunger.
5) Deposit the anaesthetic solution slowly; a slow rate of injection significantly reduces discomfort for the patient.
6) Allow the local anaesthetic sufficient time to anaesthetise the tissues, based upon the pharmacokinetic properties of the solution, and monitor the patient for any adverse reaction.

This technique can be difficult when patients have severe trismus, have a prognathic or retrognathic mandible, or are edentulous, or when there is excessive adiposity, making it difficult to locate anatomical landmarks.

If bone is contacted prematurely, then the needle is likely to be orientated too far anteriorly, against the anterior border of the ramus or temporal crest. The needle will need to be directed more posteriorly in order to deposit the anaesthesia in the correct region; that is, adjacent to the mandibular canal.

Care must be taken to not advance the needle too far posteriorly. The posterior wall of the pterygomandibular space is formed by the parotid gland, in which the motor branches of the facial

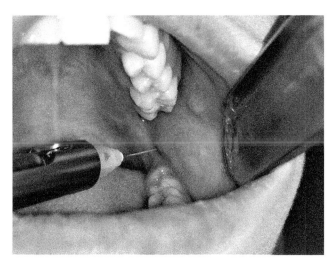

Figure 2.5   Conventional 'open-mouth' technique.

nerve course. If local anaesthetic solution is inadvertently injected into the parotid gland, the patient will develop a transient facial nerve palsy for the duration of effect of the local anaesthetic. Local anaesthetic solution should not be deposited until bony contact is noted against the needle point during insertion, confirming the correct location of the needle.

2.5.2.2   Akinosi 'Closed-Mouth' Technique

The 'closed-mouth' or Akinosi block can be utilised to anaesthetise the inferior alveolar nerve and the lingual nerve. It is useful in cases where there is severe trismus or macroglossia, or if the patient has a prominent gag reflex.

1) Position the patient in the dental chair, lying flat with head slightly extended.
2) Retract the buccal tissues to place tension on the pterygomandibular soft tissues and obtain sufficient vision and access (Figure 2.6).
3) Slowly advance the needle buccal to the maxillary molars, parallel to the occlusal plane at the level of the gingival margin of the maxillary teeth.
4) Advancing the needle in this manner, pierce the mucosa overlying the medial aspect of the mandible. Continue to advance approximately 2 cm. Because of the orientation of the needle, there is no bony anatomic landmark that will indicate the correct location of the needle tip relative to the lingula; as such, it is not recommended to insert the needle further, as the parotid space will be entered.
5) Aspirate the syringe to ensure the needle point has not traversed the intravascular space of a blood vessel.
6) Deposit the anaesthetic solution slowly; a slow rate of injection significantly reduces discomfort for the patient.
7) Allow the local anaesthetic sufficient time to anaesthetise the tissues, based upon the pharmacokinetic properties of the solution, and monitor the patient for any adverse reaction.

2.5.2.3   Gow–Gates Technique

This is a well described but technically challenging method of obtaining mandibular anaesthesia that uses extraoral landmarks to guide the needle path of insertion. It results in deposition of anaesthetic

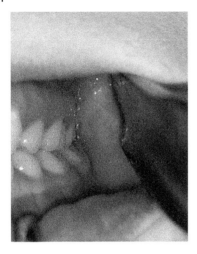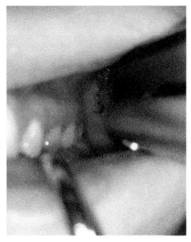

Figure 2.6 Akinosi 'closed-mouth' technique. *Source:* Seth Delpachitra.

higher in the pterygomandibular space compared with the conventional and Akinosi techniques. The benefit of a Gow–Gates block is that the inferior alveolar, lingual, and long buccal nerves may all be anaesthetised in a single injection, reducing the need for multiple anaesthetic injections.

1) Position the patient in the dental chair, lying flat with head slightly extended and mouth open.
2) Orientate the syringe and needle along an axis formed between the tragus of the ear of the side of the patient being anaesthetised and the contralateral oral commissure (Figure 2.7).
3) Place the needle tip just distobuccal to the second maxillary molar tooth (where present), and slowly advance it into the buccal mucosa in this area. The needle will advance approximately 2.5 cm before contacting the bone of the pterygoid fovea on the mandibular condyle.
4) Aspirate the syringe to ensure the needle point has not traversed the intravascular space of a blood vessel.
5) Deposit the anaesthetic solution slowly; a slow rate of injection significantly reduces discomfort for the patient.
6) Allow the local anaesthetic sufficient time to anaesthetise the tissues, based upon the pharmacokinetic properties of the solution, and monitor the patient for any adverse reaction.

2.5.2.4 Mandibular Long Buccal Block

The conventional and Akinosi block techniques do not anaesthetise the buccal mucosa of mandibular teeth; as such, in order to obtain total anaesthesia for the removal of such teeth, the buccal mucosa will need to be anaesthetised using a separate technique. The long buccal nerve is a branch of the third division of the trigeminal nerve, which travels inferoanteriorly along the condyle and external oblique ridge, descending at the anterior border of the ramus on the lateral aspect of the mandible and supplying the buccal mucosa.

1) Position the patient in the dental chair, lying flat with head slightly extended and mouth open.
2) Retract the buccal mucosa to keep the soft tissues under tension.
3) Palpate the external oblique ridge of the mandibular ramus, just posterior and lateral to the molar teeth.
4) Insert the needle into the mucosa just lateral to the external oblique ridge, to a depth of approximately 2 mm (Figure 2.8).

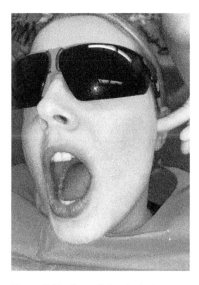
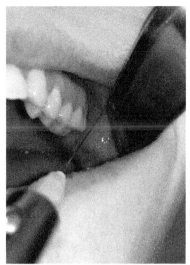

Figure 2.7   Gow–Gates technique.

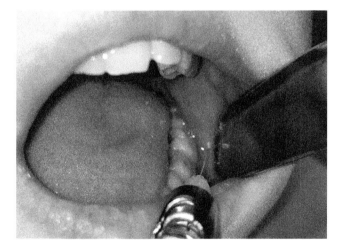

Figure 2.8   Mandibular long buccal block.

5) Aspirate the syringe to ensure the needle point has not traversed the intravascular space of a blood vessel.
6) Deposit the anaesthetic solution slowly; a slow rate of injection significantly reduces discomfort for the patient.
7) Allow the local anaesthetic sufficient time to anaesthetise the tissues, based upon the pharmacokinetic properties of the solution, and monitor the patient for any adverse reaction.

2.5.2.5   Mental Nerve Block

The mental nerve is located between the roots of the first and second premolars in the mandible, as it exits the mandible body via the mental foramen. It supplies sensation to the gingiva and mucosa anterior to the premolar region, as well as the lip and chin.

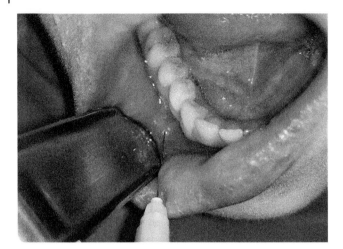

Figure 2.9   Mental nerve block.

1) Position the patient in the dental chair, lying flat with head slightly extended and mouth open.
2) Retract the labial mucosa to keep the soft tissues under tension.
3) Insert the needle into the mucosa in the deepest part of the vestibule, between the lower first and second premolar teeth, to a depth of approximately 2 mm (Figure 2.9). It is not necessary for the needle tip to contact bone for this technique to be successful.
4) Aspirate the syringe to ensure the needle point has not traversed the intravascular space of a blood vessel.
5) Deposit the anaesthetic solution slowly; a slow rate of injection significantly reduces discomfort for the patient.
6) Allow the local anaesthetic sufficient time to anaesthetise the tissues, based upon the pharmacokinetic properties of the solution, and monitor the patient for any adverse reaction.

2.5.3   Maxillary Teeth

The maxillary teeth, periodontium, and mucosa are innervated by the maxillary division of the trigeminal nerve (Figure 2.10). This nerve trunk exits the cranium via the foramen rotundum, entering the pterygopalatine fossa. One of the branches given off in the pterygopalatine fossa is the **posterior superior alveolar nerve**, which passes through the pterygomaxillary fissure into the infratemporal fossa and descends on to the posterior surface of the maxilla, before traversing forward and innervating the posterior maxillary gingiva and teeth. Branches of this nerve supply the maxillary molars, and the mucosa on the buccal aspect of those teeth.

The nerve continues to branch as it courses anteriorly, giving rise to the **middle superior alveolar nerve**, which innervates the maxillary premolars and associated buccal gingiva, and finally the **anterior superior alveolar nerve**, which innervates the maxillary incisors, canines, and associated buccal gingiva.

The **greater and lesser palatine nerves** arise from the pterygopalatine ganglion located within the pterygopalatine fossa. These nerves descend through the palatine canal. The greater palatine nerve exits on to the posterior surface of the maxilla via the greater palatine foramen and gives rise to branches which supply the palatal mucosa from the midline to the canine tooth. The lesser palatine nerve exits the lesser palatine foramen and supplies innervation to the soft palate.

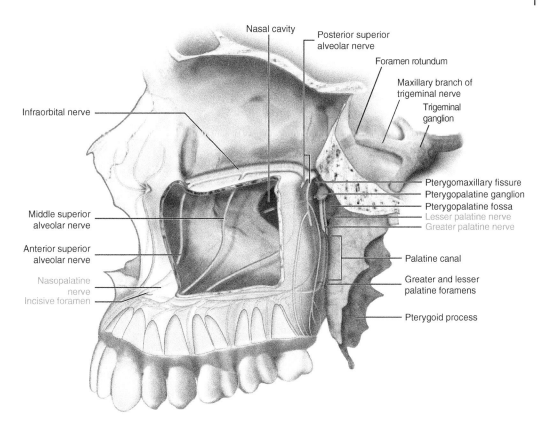

Figure 2.10   Anatomy of nerve supply to the maxilla.

The **nasopalatine nerve** travels anteriorly from the pterygopalatine ganglion through the sphenopalatine foramen, entering the nasal cavity. It travels anteriorly then inferiorly, entering the incisive canal and on to the anterior aspect of the hard palate via the incisive foramen. The nasopalatine nerve supplies the sensation to the palatal mucosa of the canines and incisors.

2.5.3.1   Greater Palatine Block

This nerve block can be used to provide anaesthesia for the palatal mucosa of the maxilla to the midline and up to the canine area. In the majority of cases, this foramen is adjacent or just distal to the second maxillary molar area.

1) Position the patient in the dental chair, lying flat with head slightly extended and mouth open.
2) Using the back end of a dental mirror or similar instrument, place pressure on the palatal mucosa adjacent to the third molar area 1–2cm medial to the gingival margin of the tooth.
3) Advance the needle into the mucosa in this region (Figure 2.11).
4) Aspirate the syringe to ensure the needle point has not traversed the intravascular space of a blood vessel.
5) Deposit the anaesthetic solution slowly; a slow rate of injection significantly reduces discomfort for the patient. Due to the keratinised nature of the palatal mucosa, only a small volume of solution can be injected into this space to produce anaesthesia.
6) Allow the local anaesthetic sufficient time to anaesthetise the tissues, based upon the pharmacokinetic properties of the solution, and monitor the patient for any adverse reaction.

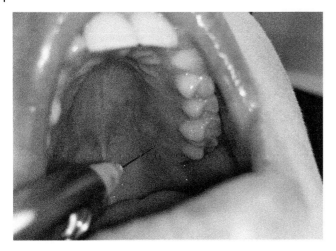

Figure 2.11   Greater palatine block.

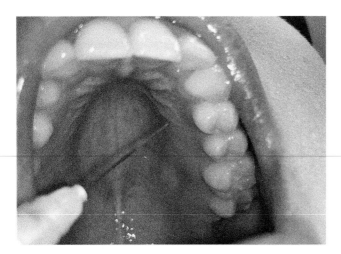

Figure 2.12   Palatal infiltration.

2.5.3.2 Palatal Infiltration

1) Position the patient in the dental chair, lying flat with head slightly extended and mouth open.
2) Using the back end of a dental mirror or similar instrument, place pressure on the palatal mucosa adjacent to the site of injection.
3) Advance the needle through the depth of the palatal mucosa, adjacent to the teeth where anaesthesia is required (Figure 2.12).
4) Aspirate the syringe to ensure the needle point has not traversed the intravascular space of a blood vessel.
5) Deposit the anaesthetic solution slowly; a slow rate of injection significantly reduces discomfort for the patient. Due to the keratinised nature of the palatal mucosa, only minute volumes of solution can be injected into the palatal mucosal to produce anaesthesia. Examine for blanching of the tissues as evidence of successful infiltration of anaesthetic solution.
6) Allow the local anaesthetic sufficient time to anaesthetise the tissues, based upon the pharmacokinetic properties of the solution, and monitor the patient for any adverse reaction.

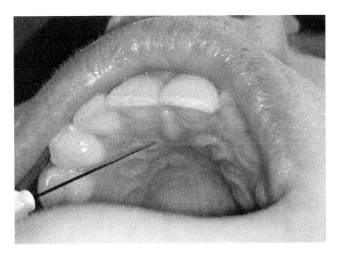

Figure 2.13   Nasopalatine nerve block. *Source:* Seth Delpachitra.

2.5.3.3   Nasopalatine Nerve Block

The nasopalatine nerve supplies sensation to the palatal gingiva posterior to the maxillary incisors and canines. This nerve can be anaesthetised by depositing local anaesthesia around the incisive papilla.

1) Position the patient in the dental chair, lying flat with head slightly extended and mouth open.
2) Locate the incisive papilla, which is often readily discernible as a raised midline structure posterior to the central incisors.
3) Insert the needle adjacent to the incisive papilla (Figure 2.13).
4) Aspirate the syringe to ensure the needle point has not traversed the intravascular space of a blood vessel.
5) Deposit the anaesthetic solution slowly; a slow rate of injection significantly reduces discomfort for the patient. Due to the keratinised nature of the palatal mucosa, only minute volumes of solution can be injected into the palatal mucosal to produce anaesthesia. Examine for blanching of the tissues as evidence of successful infiltration of anaesthetic solution.
6) Allow the local anaesthetic sufficient time to anaesthetise the tissues, based upon the pharmacokinetic properties of the solution, and monitor the patient for any adverse reaction.

2.5.3.4   Posterior Superior Alveolar Nerve Block

If anaesthesia of the hemimaxilla is required (e.g. in a full maxillary dental clearance), a posterior superior alveolar nerve block may be used in lieu of multiple buccal infiltration anaesthetics. This technique is not dissimilar to conventional buccal infiltration; the major difference is that the location of anaesthetic solution deposition is in the infratemporal fossa just behind the posterior maxilla, where the posterior superior alveolar nerve trunk travels.

1) Position the patient in the dental chair, lying flat with head slightly extended and mouth slightly open.
2) Palpate the zygomatic buttress and take note of its relative position, usually just superior to the first or second maxillary molar.
3) Retract the buccal tissues, such that the buccal gingiva, maxillary tuberosity, and cervical margin of the maxillary teeth can be visualised and the buccal soft tissues are taut.

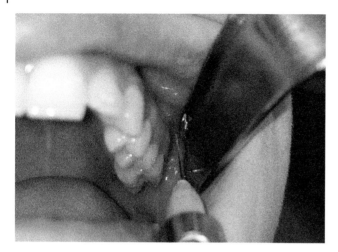

Figure 2.14 Posterior superior alveolar nerve block.

4) Insert the needle into the vestibular mucosa just posterior to the maxillary tuberosity, angled at 45° to the occlusal plane (Figure 2.14). Advance it approximately 1–1.5 cm.
5) Aspirate the syringe to ensure the needle point has not traversed the intravascular space of a blood vessel.
6) Deposit the anaesthetic solution slowly; a slow rate of injection significantly reduces discomfort for the patient.
7) Allow the local anaesthetic sufficient time to anaesthetise the tissues, based upon the pharmacokinetic properties of the solution, and monitor the patient for any adverse reaction.

2.6 Adjunct Methods of Local Anaesthesia

In certain situations of dental extraction, it may be difficult to obtain complete anaesthesia using the standard infiltration and block techniques described in the previous section. The following methods may be utilised if additional anaesthesia of a single tooth is required mid-procedure. Note that they cannot be used alone to obtain sufficient anaesthesia for dental extraction.

2.6.1 Intraligamentary Injection

1) Advance a short needle into the periodontal ligament space. The needle should be felt to 'wedge' into the space between tooth and bone; this is required to ensure the anaesthetic solution is delivered into the correct site.
2) Deposit the anaesthesia. Firm pressure on the syringe will be required to deposit the solution. Due to the extremely small periodontal ligament space, only minute volumes of solution can be injected using this technique.
3) Repeat in at least four positions around the tooth.
4) Allow the local anaesthetic sufficient time to anaesthetise the tissues, based upon the pharmacokinetic properties of the solution, and monitor the patient for any adverse reaction.

2.6.2 Intrapulpal Injection

Intrapulpal injection is useful in cases where an attempt to section a tooth has already been made and the patient has experienced pain during instrumenting or sectioning. As the name suggests, the anaesthetic agent is injected into the pulp chamber to directly anaesthetise the pulpal tissues.

1) Position the patient in the dental chair, allowing for adequate light and access to the dental pulp.
2) Visualise the pulp chamber – this will be the site of needle entry.
3) Advance a short needle into the pulp chamber (Figure 2.15).
4) Deposit local anaesthetic into the pulp. As the volume of the pulp chamber is small, only a minute volume of anaesthetic is required to achieve pulpal anaesthesia. It may be necessary to apply firm pressure on the syringe in order to deliver the solution into the chamber.
5) Allow the local anaesthetic sufficient time to anaesthetise the tissues, based upon the pharmacokinetic properties of the solution, and monitor the patient for any adverse reaction.

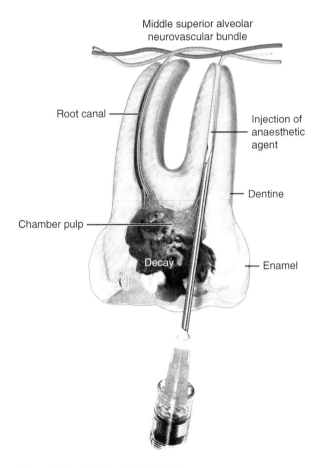

Figure 2.15 Intrapulpal injection.

2.7 Troubleshooting

The goal of injecting local anaesthesia is to prevent the patient from perceiving pain when tissues are manipulated. There are a number of reasons why anaesthetic may fail, although the majority of cases are due to poor technique:

- Anxiety and dental fear by the patient.
- Local inflammatory conditions or the pulp or surrounding tissues.
- Variations in local anatomy.
- Accessory innervation of the teeth or surrounding structures.
- Thick cortical bone preventing diffusion.
- Inadequate dose for the procedure.
- Inadequate time for onset of anaesthetic effect.

A common misconception amongst patients undergoing procedures with local anaesthesia is that they will feel nothing. If patients are not sufficiently informed that anaesthesia only inhibits local pain signalling, they may perceive the sensation of pushing forces on the jaws as failed anaesthesia. Anxiety and dental fear can also heighten the experience of pain and otherwise innocuous stimuli. Patients should be informed that whilst profound anaesthesia can inhibit local pain signalling, this does not extend to reducing pressure on the entire mandible and maxilla. If, despite forewarning, the patient still does not tolerate the procedure, additional forms of anaesthesia may be indicated.

Inadequate anaesthesia may also be related to improper technique or variations in anatomy. When administering an inferior alveolar nerve block, there are a number of anatomical variants which can lead to failed anaesthesia. A flared ramus, accessory mandibular foramen, or abnormal position of the mandibular foramen may prevent the block from being effective. Failure of an infiltration anaesthetic may also be due to local anatomical factors, such as a thick cortical plate or exostosis limiting the diffusion of the anaesthetic agent.

In some cases, mandibular teeth may receive accessory sensory innervation by the nerve to mylohyoid. This nerve branches from the inferior alveolar nerve before it enters the mandibular foramen. Its primary function is as a motor nerve to the mylohyoid muscle, but it may also carry sensory fibres, which can provide innervation to mandibular molars. As this nerve branches higher in the pterygomandibular space, a traditional inferior alveolar nerve block may not adequately anaesthetise the mandibular teeth. In such cases – where the operator is assured that the lower lip and chin are anaesthetised, and adequate buccal anaesthesia has been obtained – additional local anaesthesia in the form of intraligamental injections may be used to account for this anatomic variant.

Localised infections, dental abscesses, and inflammatory oedema can significantly reduce the efficacy of local anaesthetic. In solution, local anaesthetic molecules exist in both ionised form, which cannot cross nerve membranes, and unionised form, which can. Tissues undergoing an inflammatory or infectious process may be more acidic, increasing the proportion of injected anaesthetic molecules that are ionised versus unionised. Less of the solution will effectively block the voltage-gated sodium channels, and its anaesthetic effect will thus be reduced. Use of buffered anaesthetic agents containing bicarbonate allows for less ionisation and therefore more effective anaesthesia.

Inflammatory conditions of the pulpal tissues, or 'hot pulp', can also lead to a failure to adequately anaesthetise the tooth, through hyperalgesia and nerve sensitisation due to the presence of inflammatory mediators. In these situations, additional forms of anaesthesia may be required for patient comfort.

An inadequate dose is another common reason for failure. For general and restorative dentistry, an approach of using as little anaesthesia as possible is generally favoured. The advantage from the patient's perspective is that the lack of sensation is shorter in duration, there is less chance of producing tachycardia, and fewer injections are required. However, when using local anaesthesia for dentoalveolar extractions, more profound anaesthesia is required, and the clinician should bear this in mind when planning dose and delivery. The anaesthetic technique must ensure that the tissues are sufficiently anaesthetised and that the patient has sufficient time after the procedure to commence analgesics before the local anaesthetic effect wears off.

3

Basic Surgical Instruments

A complete surgical instrument tray is essential to safely and effectively perform dentoalveolar extractions. Every piece of equipment on the surgical setup serves a specific role in the removal of a tooth from the oral cavity. An understanding of the correct indications, uses, and limitations of each is therefore paramount in reducing the risk of failed extraction or prolonged operating time. Whilst a great range of instruments are available, a basic set is usually sufficient, awareness of which can save the surgeon significant practice costs. This chapter introduces the various tools one should be familiar with in an oral surgical practice, outlining their names, indications, and instructions for use.

As with any surgical procedure, adequate pre-planning is paramount when undertaking dentoalveolar extractions to ensure that the surgeon has all equipment ready and within easy reach, and to reduce delays in completion. This is particularly important for extractions under local anaesthetic, where both appropriate use of instruments and minimisation of operative time can significantly improve patient comfort and tolerance.

Broadly, surgical instruments for dental extraction can be categorised as follows:

- **Retractors.** Instruments used to displace tissues and improve surgical access.
- **Elevators, Luxators, and Periotomes.** Shanked instruments used to disrupt the periodontal ligament and mobilise teeth against the bony socket.
- **Extraction Forceps.** Pincer-type instruments used to grasp, mobilise, and deliver teeth or roots.
- **Ancillary Soft Tissue Instruments.** Additional instruments used during and after dental extraction, to manipulate the soft tissues.
- **Suturing Equipment.** Specialised equipment necessary for the handling of a suture needle and soft tissues, for wound closure.
- **Surgical Suction and Irrigation.** Suction and irrigation devices that can be safely and effectively used in a surgical site.
- **Surgical Handpieces and Burs.** Drills designed specifically for use in dentoalveolar surgery.

3.1 Retractors

The **Cawood-Minnesota retractor** is a versatile instrument used by the surgeon during surgical extraction procedures (Figure 3.1). It is broad and flat, with one curved end, which can be used as a lip retractor, and one flat, pointed end, which is usually used to retract mucoperiosteal flaps. It is held in the nondominant hand, with the index and middle fingers on the front of the instrument

Principles of Dentoalveolar Extractions, First Edition. Seth Delpachitra, Anton Sklavos and Ricky Kumar.
© 2021 John Wiley & Sons Ltd. Published 2021 by John Wiley & Sons Ltd.
Companion website: www.wiley.com/go/delpachitradentoalveolarextractions

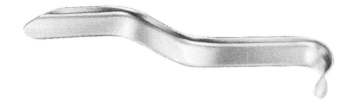

Figure 3.1 Cawood-Minnesota retractor. Only a gentle finger grip is required in its use. Excessive grip strength reduces tactile feedback from the instrument, can strain the operator's hand, and can lead to unnecessary soft tissue injury from the sharp tip of the retractor. *Source:* KLS Martin.

and the thumb positioned directly behind the fingers on the back. The sharp end should only be pressed against hard tissues, as excessive downward force against soft tissues can lead to mucosal or gingival lacerations.

A **wire cheek retractor** is used by the surgical assistant during oral surgical procedures, to retract the lips and improve surgical access (Figure 3.2). It is named for its construction from a heavy-gauge, stainless-steel wire that has been twisted to produce a curved retractor on either end. It is particularly useful during suturing, when the primary operator's hands are both in use.

A **tongue retractor** is used only during general anaesthetic cases (Figure 3.3). It has a large, broad blade attached at 90° to the handle. It is excellent for displacement of the lingual soft tissues to improve surgical access, but is very uncomfortable for the awake patient, and can initiate a gag reflex.

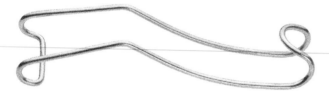

Figure 3.2 Wire cheek retractor. This instrument is most commonly held by the surgeon's assistant. One major limitation is its propensity to slip away from the oral cavity whilst in use. Holding it in the palm of the hand, with a gentle grip, and an outward and downward direction, helps to engage the lip and cheek and reduce retractor slippage. *Source:* KLS Martin.

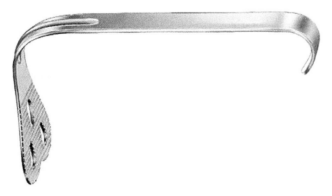

Figure 3.3 Tongue retractor. This instrument is large and can damage the anterior teeth if used incorrectly. It should be inserted such that the blade is parallel to the occlusal plane; once inside the oral cavity, it may be rotated 90° to rest against the tongue. *Source:* KLS Martin.

3.2 Elevators, Luxators, and Periotomes

These exist within a group of instruments designed to apply unidirectional force on to a tooth. This force is generally used initially to break the periodontal ligament, but on specific occasions it is sufficient to completely dislodge a tooth from its supporting tissues. All elevators have the same basic construction (Figure 3.4).

The **handle** is designed to fit ergonomically into the palm and fingers of the operator's hand. A number of types of handle are available, deliberately designed based on how much force the tip of the instrument can safely apply to the hard tissues. T-type handles have fallen out of favour in the contemporary basic set of instruments, because of their potential to exert excessive force on tooth and bone, resulting in injury.

The **shank** is the intermediate bar between the handle and the tip of the elevator. It may be straight or angled, depending on the function of the instrument. A shorter shank can improve instrument handling but limit access to the posterior teeth; conversely, a longer shank may be more difficult to control but has better access.

The **tip** is the major component that defines the elevator's function. A large variety of tips exist, each serving a different purpose. A thin, flatter tip, such as that of a fine luxator, is indicated for wedging between tooth and bone, to disrupt the periodontal ligament. The curved, blunt tip of a Warwick-James is particularly useful for upper third molar teeth, providing a distobuccal tipping force, and guiding the tooth along its root axis. A sharp, pointed tip such as is seen on a Cryer elevator is designed to wedge into a point of elevation on the lateral surface of a tooth root and provide a strong apico-coronal force.

Three biomechanical principles can be applied when using elevators (Figure 3.5):

- **Wedging** is the use of an instrument with a sharply acute angle to split or divide objects using a downward force. This is the common use of a periotome or luxator to widen the periodontal ligament space. Whilst use of a wedging force can be the best way to initiate breaking of the

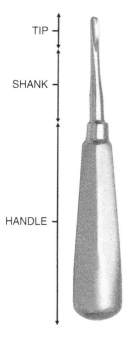

TIP

SHANK

HANDLE

Figure 3.4 Basic elevator construction.

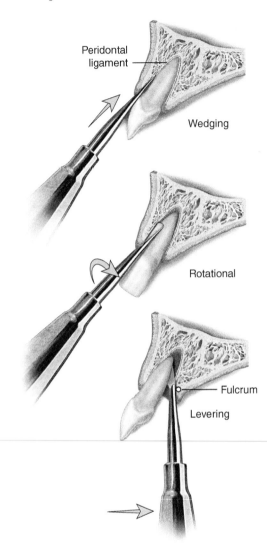

Figure 3.5   Types of forces applicable through an elevator.

periodontal ligament, extreme care should be taken with regard to the amount of force placed along the instrument, as slippage of a sharp elevator due to uncontrolled pressure along its axis can very quickly and easily lead to significant soft tissue injuries.

- **Rotational** movements involve the rotational force of an instrument along its axis, to apply a torque force through the tip. This is the most common biomechanical use of elevators. Whilst rotation of an instrument is a relatively safe manoeuvre, it must be kept in mind that a rotating elevator has two points of force propagation (at the end of the tip and at the instrument axis), and the bone being elevated against must be of sufficient strength to withstand the opposing force. Excessive rotational force against weak mandibular bone may result in mandibular fracture, a catastrophic outcome. Similarly, the force placed against the tooth being extracted will not always be along its strongest axis, and this may result in tooth fracture mid-extraction.
- **Levering** involves positioning the tip of an elevator such that the handle and tip lie on either side of a fulcrum, formed between the shank of the instrument and the alveolar bone. A lever

Table 3.1 General principles of elevator use.

1) Avoid excessive, uncontrolled forces during levering, rotation, or wedging.
2) Do not luxate between teeth – only between tooth and stable alveolar bone.
3) Use the correct instrument, in the correct way, for the correct indication.
4) Ensure a stable purchase point on the tooth being extracted, to which the elevator can engage.
5) Use the fingers of the nondominant hand as a protective mechanism, holding the buccal and lingual/palatal plates of the alveolus to buffer against instrument slippage and balance against excessive force.

motion enables an upward direction of force against a tooth root and can allow elevation out of the socket. Use of the levering motion should be avoided where possible, however, as two critical failures may occur. First, it places undue perpendicular mechanical stress against the shank of the instrument, which may result in instrument breakage. Second, the fulcrum point of shank against bone will undoubtedly damage the thin alveolus of the periodontium, compromising socket healing.

The basic principles of elevator use are described in Table 3.1.

Common types of elevators and their indications are listed in Table 3.2.

Table 3.2 Common elevator designs and indications for use. Image *source:* KLS Martin.

Elevator	Image	Features	Uses
Luxator/periotome	5,0 mm	Straight shank Sharp, curved tip Available in various widths (3 mm, 5 mm)	Disruption of periodontal ligament Expansion of alveolar socket Gentle mobilisation of tooth Elevation of tooth roots
Coupland's No. 2 Gouge	2,5 mm	Straight shank Blunt, curved tip	Mobilisation of teeth

(Continued)

Table 3.2 (Continued)

Elevator	Image		Features	Uses
Cryer (Left, Right)	8,2 mm	8,2 mm	Angled, triangular tip with sharp end	Gripping a point of application on a tooth to provide strong directional force
Warwick-James (Left, Right)	2,2 mm	2,2 mm	Angled, curved, rounded 'golf club' tip	Gripping a point of application on a tooth to provide moderate directional force
Root Pick			Thin, angled shank	Access to apical areas of fractured roots to manoeuvre between bone and tooth root, in order to deliver a light extraction force
			Small, sharp, straight tip with slight curvature	

3.3 Dental Extraction Forceps

Forceps are the cornerstone instrument of dental extractions. When applied and used correctly, they can simultaneously provide the wedging force of an elevator between tooth and bone, allow for slow expansion of the bony socket, mobilise the tooth along its strongest axis, and grasp and deliver the tooth.

This multifunctional application can lead to difficulty in the use of a forceps – there must be a harmonious balance between the squeezing, twisting, and levering forces that are applied through the instrument, and each type of force must be used at the correct magnitude and in the correct stage of an extraction. For example, applying too firm a grip on the tooth early in the process can cause crown fracture, necessitating a switch to surgical extraction methods. Similarly, applying a twisting force without sufficient grip leads to inefficient use of the instrument and considerable difficulty in mobilising the tooth. This balance of forces can only be developed with time, practice, and close attention to the effect of the instrument on the hard tissues.

Like elevators, all dental extraction forceps have the same basic construction. Generally, forceps resemble a set of short-nosed pliers (Figure 3.6).

The **handle** is long and usually textured, and is designed to be gripped in the palm, secured with the thumb on one side and four fingers on the other. This design allows the operator to apply maximum grip strength on the handle in order to transmit this force to the beaks and tooth. The handle is longer than the beaks, allowing for magnification of forces applied around the tooth axis when using a rotatory motion.

The **hinge** is the mechanical joint that allows the extraction forceps to open and close. Inadequate maintenance of forceps over time may lead to loosening of the hinge, reducing the efficacy of the instrument. **British pattern** forceps have a hinge directed horizontally to the handle, whilst **American pattern** forceps have a hinge directed vertically. Although the beaks of each pattern are similar, the hinge orientation may alter the direction of force applied through the forceps.

The **beaks** are the most important variable component of the dental extraction forceps. Conceptually, each concave beak should be considered as an elevator, as sharp, and as purpose-designed to wrap around one aspect of a tooth's root surface. The beaks, when used together, should therefore almost exactly wrap around the tooth's cementoenamel junction. Beaks may lie at

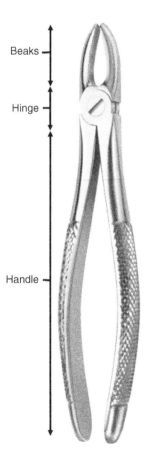

Beaks

Hinge

Handle

Figure 3.6   Basic forceps construction.

Table 3.3   General principles of dental extraction forceps use.

1) Choose the correct forceps for the task at hand, based upon beak shape and contour.
2) Hold the instrument correctly, using the palm of the hand, and stand in the correct position to maximise the biomechanics of the shoulder and elbow.
3) Apply the forceps to the tooth in such a way that the maximum surface area of the beaks is against the cementoenamel junction.
4) Balance the wedging, rotational, and levering forces appropriately.

the same axis as the handle, or with an angle of up to 90 degrees, depending on the purpose of the instrument and the tooth location for which it is designed. Choosing the correct forceps for a dental extraction is therefore entirely dependent on the beak design; that is, the type of beak that will best match the root structure of the tooth, and the angulation that will best allow for biomechanical advantage depending on the location of the tooth in the mouth and the patient position.

The basic principles of forceps use are described in Table 3.3.

There are a large variety of dental extraction forceps available, with different beaks and angle orientations, as shown in Table 3.4.

Table 3.4   Common dental extraction forceps designs (American and British patterns). Image *source:* KLS Martin.

Elevator	American pattern	British pattern
Upper Straight	3,0 mm	3,2 mm
Upper Universal	2,6 mm	4,6 mm

Table 3.4   (Continued)

Elevator	American pattern	British pattern
Upper Molar (Left)	6,1 mm	7,6 mm
Upper Molar (Right)		7,6 mm
Lower Universal	4,3 mm	3,1 mm
Lower Hawk	7,0 mm	5,9 mm
Cowhorn	16,5 mm	1,8 mm

3.4 Ancillary Soft Tissue Instruments

The process of dental extraction often involves more than just tooth removal. Prior to removal, manipulation of the soft tissues may be necessary to gain sufficient access before elevators or forceps can be applied to a tooth. Following removal, there may be debris or pathology within the socket that requires debridement or removal to ensure satisfactory postoperative healing.

The **scalpel** is the main instrument used to cut the fine periodontal soft tissues of the oral cavity (Figure 3.7). A key consideration in the selection of cutting instruments for use in the oral cavity is the need to maintain control over them, as larger instruments may cause damage to the surrounding perioral tissues such as the lips and cheeks. Whilst a large variety of scalpel handle and blade configurations are available, a No. 3 or No. 7 handle with a 15 blade affords good instrument control and safe application in the mouth.

A **periosteal elevator** is used to lift a mucoperiosteal flap off the bone, either to facilitate access to the subgingival root of the tooth or to visualise the alveolar bone prior to removal. Whilst many designs are available, the Molt elevator is the most versatile for use in the oral cavity (Figure 3.8). It is designed with one sharp, pointed end and one flat, curved, 'beaver-tail' end, and is useful for elevating crestal gingiva.

The **Mitchell's trimmer** was historically intended as a crown-preparation instrument in dentistry, but now is more commonly used in minor oral surgery as an instrument of soft tissue curettage (Figure 3.9). It is a double-ended instrument on a shank; one end is spoon-shaped, and is small enough to enucleate periapical cysts or remove debris from a tooth socket, whilst the other is a tapered, right-angled point, and can be used for curettage or for removal of sharp alveolar bone edges.

An **angled curette** is a common, double-ended surgical instrument with two curettes at opposite angles to one another which can be used in a similar fashion as a Mitchell's trimmer to debride sockets or enucleate periapical cysts (Figure 3.10). Angled curettes are relatively unlikely to be found in a basic dentoalveolar set, as their function is largely met by the Mitchell's trimmer.

A **cleoid-discoid carver** is another instrument of restorative dentistry that has become a feature of dentoalveolar surgical setups (Figure 3.11). This fine, double-ended instrument has a

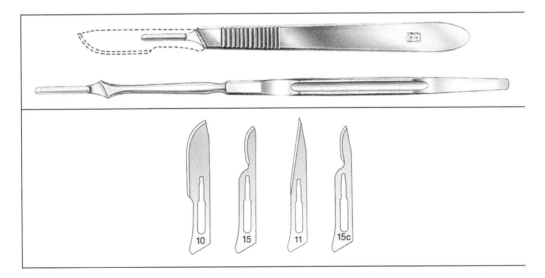

Figure 3.7 Scalpel handle and blade types commonly used in dentoalveolar surgery. *Source:* KLS Martin.

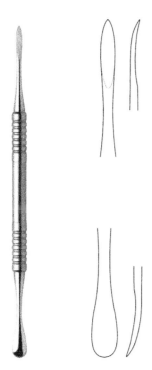

Figure 3.8   Molt periosteal elevator. Each end has two surfaces: one rounded and one relatively flat. The round surface should be directed towards the soft tissue, whilst the flat, sharp surface should be directed towards the alveolar bone. The pointed end can be used to retract the interdental papilla, which makes raising a full-thickness mucoperiosteal flap much easier and limits tearing of the flap due to cleavage in a supraperiosteal plane. *Source:* KLS Martin.

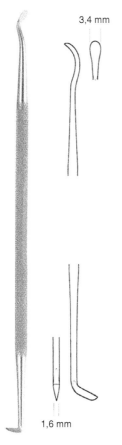

3,4 mm

1,6 mm

Figure 3.9   Mitchell's trimmer. *Source:* Laurence Jordan, Francois Bronnec, Pierre Machtou.

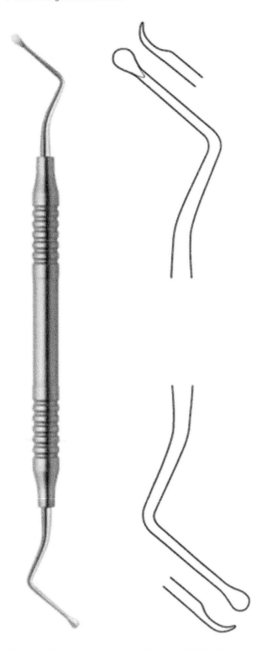

Figure 3.10   Angled curette. *Source:* KLS Martin.

leaf-shaped ('cleoid') element and a disc-shaped ('discoid') element. It is ideal for access to and debridement of the restricted apical areas of the tooth socket, where other curettage instruments may be too large.

Curved artery forceps are an all-purpose grasping instrument, used to remove loose bone or tooth fragments from a socket (Figure 3.12). The end of the instrument is blunt and curved, with a serrated working surface.

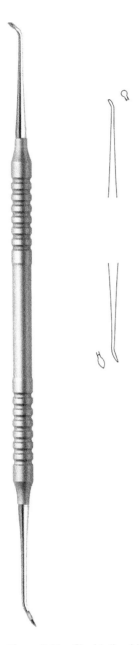

Figure 3.11   Cleoid-discoid carver. *Source:* KLS Martin.

3.5   Suturing Instruments

During removal of a tooth, the soft tissues may be intentionally or inadvertently compromised. Instruments for the manipulation and suturing of soft tissues thus form an important part of a basic oral surgical setup (Figure 3.13). This is a very common requirement after extraction of multiple teeth or surgical extraction, or in medically compromised patients where good wound closure or haemostasis is critical.

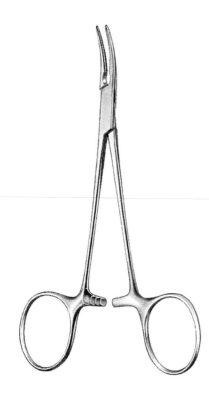

Figure 3.12   Curved artery forceps. *Source:* KLS Martin.

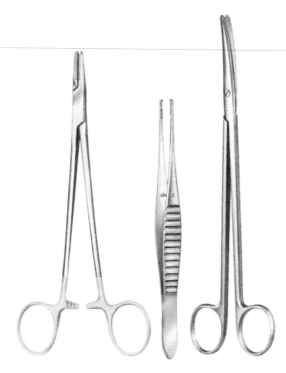

Figure 3.13   Basic suturing equipment. Needle holders, forceps, and scissors come in a variety of sizes. As dentoalveolar surgery is carried out in the confines of the patient's mouth, larger instruments make it more difficult to access the posterior aspects. Small needle holders with a fine tip offer good manoeuvrability and control of the soft tissues. *Source:* KLS Martin.

Needle-holding forceps are purpose-built instruments, important features of which include:

- A finger-ring handle design, for easy manoeuvrability in the oral cavity.
- A ratchet, to allow the instrument to keep a fixed suture needle position without application of force.
- A cross-hatched working surface, to allow the holding of a suture needle across a broad range of angulations.

These instruments allow for correct use of a suture needle, reducing the propensity for soft tissue trauma from excessive manipulation of the friable mucosa and gingiva. The most common design used in oral surgery is the Mayo-Hegar needle holder. A critical error made by the novice dentoalveolar surgeon is to use artery forceps instead, in order to avoid the additional cost of purchasing a needle-holding instrument. This is dangerous, as artery forceps do not provide sufficient grip or control of the suture needle, which can lead to needle breakage or poor control when working in the oral cavity.

Gilles forceps are the instrument of choice for grasping periodontal tissues to assist with approximation and closure with sutures. They are ideal for the oral cavity given their straight profile, small size, narrow jaws, and cross-serrated tips, with teeth that can hold and grip the smooth and often lubricated periodontal tissues. Gilles forceps are held in a similar manner to a pen, with the thumb and forefinger controlling the tips of the instrument.

Whilst there is no particular scissor designed for suture cutting in the oral cavity, an appropriate **suture scissor** should have sufficient handle length to access the posterior oral cavity, short blades to avoid inadvertent damage to oral tissues, and a slight curve in the blade to facilitate visualisation of the suture being cut.

Sutures are available in a wide variety of materials, needle types, and sizes (Table 3.5). Generally, suture materials are classified based upon type of material (synthetic versus natural), ability to be resorbed by the tissues, size, and structure (monofilament versus braided). Whilst the type of suture used is largely dependent on surgeon preference, each characteristic has a significant effect on intraoperative handling and postoperative healing (Table 3.6). A mid-sized (3-0 or 4-0) resorbable suture on a 3/8″ circle needle is generally acceptable for use in minor dentoalveolar surgery (Figure 3.14).

3.6 Surgical Suction

A good surgical suction device is an essential component of any dental extraction procedure, not only to provide access and visibility, but also as an important safety measure for emergency airway management. A fine (2 mm-diameter) Frasier-style suction tip, attached to a high-volume suction outlet, affords excellent manoeuvrability in the mouth and allows for rapid evacuation of surgical-site debris and fluid by the surgical assistant (Figure 3.15). Conventional low- and high-volume suction devices used in dentistry are not fit for the purpose of dentoalveolar surgery.

Table 3.5 Common suture materials used in the oral cavity, classified by behaviour and filament type.

Suture materials						
Resorbable				Nonresorbable		
Monofilament		Braided		Monofilament		Braided
Gut (plain or chromic)	Poligecaprone 25	Polyglactin 910	Polyglactin 910 (rapid)	Nylon	Polypropylene	Silk Polyester

Table 3.6 Characteristics of suture needles and materials.

Characteristic	Types	Effect on handling
Needle size	Suture needles may come in a variety of sizes, measured by the chord length between the tip and the swage	A smaller needle may be easier to manoeuvre in the oral cavity but more susceptible to deformation or breakage
Needle shape	The shape of a suture needle is based on what proportion of a full circle its arc forms, expressed as a fraction; most commonly, needles arc 1/2 or 3/8 arc	The arc of a needle affects intraoperative handling; a greater arc may help take deeper tissue bites, but is harder to manoeuvre in smaller spaces
Filament type	Monofilament	Smooth monofilaments pass through the tissues easily and do not elicit as great a tissue reaction, but are more difficult to tie due to knot slippage
	Braided	Rope-like braided filaments have better grip against tissues and are easy to tie, but may elicit a tissue reaction
Filament material	Natural	Natural filaments are degraded by proteolysis; a tissue reaction is more likely
	Synthetic	Synthetic filaments are degraded by enzymatic breakdown; a tissue reaction is less likely
Absorbability	Absorbable	Absorbable sutures do not require secondary removal, but their duration of strength may be variable
	Nonabsorbable	Nonabsorbable sutures require removal at a later stage, but their strength and hold are almost guaranteed during this time

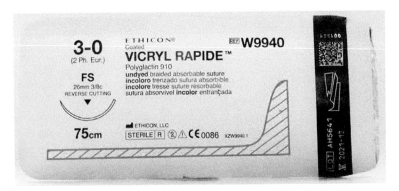

Figure 3.14 Front of a suture packet, detailing suture gauge (3-0), needle type (FS-2), shape (3/8c), suture length (75 cm), and suture material (Polyglactin 910). Also provided are an illustration, description ('undyed braided absorbable suture'), and expiration date. *Source:* Laurence Jordan, Francois Bronnec, Pierre Machtou.

3.7 Surgical Handpiece and Bur

Conventional dental high- and slow-speed handpieces are typically not suitable for dentoalveolar surgery, for several reasons:

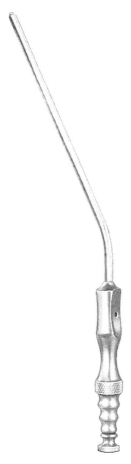

Figure 3.15   Frasier suction tip. *Source:* KLS Martin.

- Air-driven, high-speed handpieces used in dentistry are generally designed with a 'front-end' exhaust system; that is, air pressure is released axially near the bur. Use of this type of system under or near periodontal flaps and bone can push large amounts of air and coolant into the soft tissues of the head and neck, resulting in surgical emphysema.
- Slow-speed handpieces do not turn at a sufficient speed or torque to efficiently section a tooth through the enamel and dentine in a controlled fashion.
- Contra-angle handpieces may be used, but in posterior areas their head can limit visualisation of structures.

There are several components to a surgical unit: the unit itself, which allows manipulation of the torque and speed; the motor, which is usually a separate component and can be sterilised; and either a foot pedal or an attachment on the handpiece itself, to control the instrument (Figure 3.16).

3.8   Surgical Irrigation Systems

Irrigation of a surgical site with sterile saline reduces the amount of remaining debris, may improve healing, and reduce rates of postoperative infection. An efficient suction/irrigation system is also

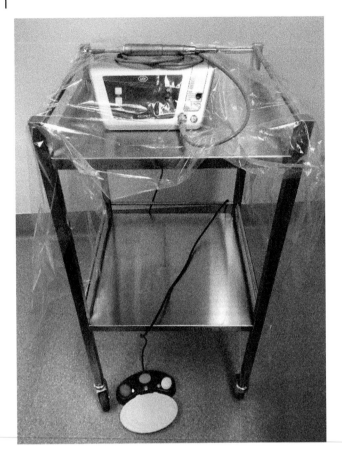

Figure 3.16 Surgical bur setup with sterile plastic and foot pedal.

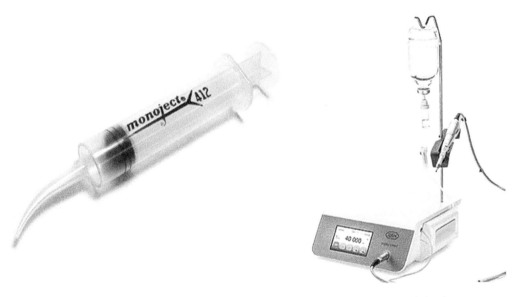

Figure 3.17 Options for surgical irrigation include use of a Monoject (R) syringe or an irrigation system inbuilt into the surgical drill. *Source:* Laurence Jordan, Francois Bronnec, Pierre Machtou.

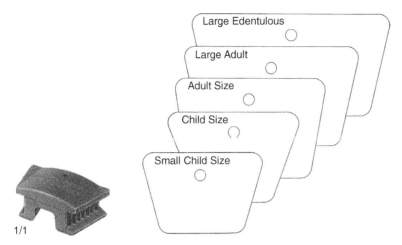

Figure 3.18 Mouth prop. A number of sizes are available. *Source:* KLS Martin.

critical when using surgical burs, as a coolant to prevent thermal osteonecrosis of the bone. In surgical situations, conventional dental unit water lines for irrigation are not suitable, as nonsterile, pressurised irrigation solutions may predispose to infection of the wound.

Some surgical handpieces come equipped to accommodate a saline bag, which will deliver the saline at the surgical handpiece tip as a coolant. Alternatively, a simple method is the use of a Monoject syringe with sterile saline solution (Figure 3.17).

3.9 Mouth Props

Application of a mouth prop is a useful safety and behaviour-modification technique (Figure 3.18). It allows the patient to keep their mouth open without active effort, and reduces the likelihood of inadvertent mouth closure whilst sharp instruments are inside. Whilst a mouth prop is only absolutely indicated for cases under general anaesthetic, its use in awake patients improves surgical access, stabilises the jaws, and reduces inadvertent swallowing by the patient.

4

Simple Extraction Techniques

This chapter discusses the specific techniques for extraction of individual teeth in the maxillary and mandibular arch in a detailed, step-wise format. Surgical extractions and third molars are discussed in the subsequent chapters.

4.1   Maxillary Incisors

1) **Difficulty Assessment.** Single-rooted maxillary incisor teeth have largely straight roots, with a slight distal curvature (Figure 4.1). Rarely, this curvature can be significant enough at the tooth apex to warrant a surgical extraction approach. This can be readily assessed on plain-film imaging.

2) **Obtain Consent.** The general risks of dental extraction apply for maxillary incisors. Any prosthetic rehabilitation plan for anterior teeth should be included in the consent process.

3) **Basic Equipment Required.** An upper straight forceps can be used for maxillary central and lateral incisors. A straight elevator should be available to expand the periodontal ligament prior to forceps placement.

4) **Final Check.** Confirm the tooth number and location with radiograph.

5) **Local Anaesthetic.** Infiltration of the buccal vestibule will provide sufficient anaesthesia for the maxillary buccal soft tissue and periodontal ligament. Localised palatal infiltration is required to anaesthetise the palatal gingiva.

6) **Positioning.** Lie the patient flat, with the maxillary teeth at the same vertical height as the surgeon's elbow. Stand on the side of the patient that corresponds with the hand dominance of the surgeon. For example, a right-handed practitioner standing on the right side of the patient increases biomechanical advantage when removing the tooth.

7) **Elevation.** Apply the straight elevator to the mesial and distal areas of the periodontal ligament. Using a wheel-and-axle motion, gently expand the periodontal ligament until a small amount of mobility is noted in the tooth. Take care to elevate between tooth and bone only, and not against adjacent teeth. The thumb and finger of the nondominant hand should be used to support the alveolus of the tooth being extracted, to guide the application of force to the tooth socket only, and to prevent instrument slippage.

Principles of Dentoalveolar Extractions, First Edition. Seth Delpachitra, Anton Sklavos and Ricky Kumar.
© 2021 John Wiley & Sons Ltd. Published 2021 by John Wiley & Sons Ltd.
Companion website: www.wiley.com/go/delpachitradentoalveolarextractions

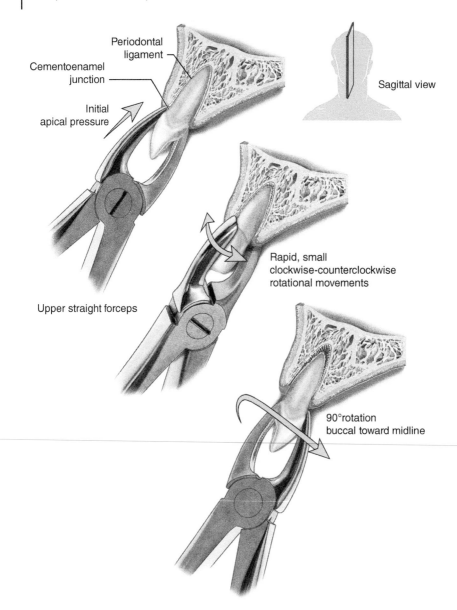

Periodontal ligament

Cementoenamel junction

Initial apical pressure

Sagittal view

Upper straight forceps

Rapid, small clockwise-counterclockwise rotational movements

90°rotation buccal toward midline

Figure 4.1 Extraction of a maxillary incisor tooth.

8) **Delivery.** Apply the beaks of the straight forceps on to the cementoenamel junction of the tooth. Initially, use apical pressure to slide the beaks as deep on to the root as possible. Employ rapid, small clockwise–counterclockwise rotational movements to continue tearing the periodontal ligament. Finally, rotate the buccal part of the crown towards the midline. This final movement reduces the risk of fracture of the curved root tip, as anterior maxillary alveolar bone is more pliable than thick palatal bone.

9) **Assessment.** Assess the tooth root to ensure it has been removed complete. Flush the socket with saline to remove any surgical debris. Examine the socket for bleeding, alveolar bone fracture, or soft tissue trauma, and manage as appropriate.

4.2   Maxillary Canines

1) **Difficulty Assessment.** Removal of the maxillary canine can often be more difficult than expected for the novice dentoalveolar surgeon due to the deceptive straight, single root (Figure 4.2). First, maxillary canines have a significantly larger periodontal surface area than maxillary incisors due to the longer root structure. Second, the buccal bone overlying the maxillary incisor may be thick and unforgiving – this can be assessed clinically by running one gloved finger over the alveolar bone and mucosa in the area. Third, maxillary canines undergo millions of cycles of repetitive and heavy lateral loading, and this can cause ankylosis or a reduced periodontal ligament space. Difficulty significantly increases when any of these three factors is seen.

2) **Obtain Consent.** In addition to the general risks of dental extraction, patients should be specifically informed of the risk of buccal alveolar fracture, as this can be common with removal of canines, and can affect future prosthetic rehabilitation.

3) **Basic Equipment Required.** Short-beaked upper straight forceps, sometimes referred to as 'stubbie' forceps, are the gold standard for removing upper canine teeth, as the shorter beak allows for greater grip force to be applied to the canine. Upper straight forceps can be used, but their thinner, longer beaks may not provide sufficient force to the tooth. A straight elevator should be available to expand the periodontal ligament prior to forceps placement.

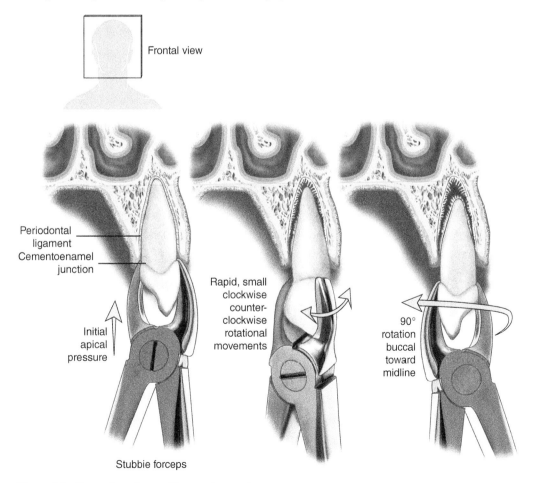

Frontal view

Periodontal ligament
Cementoenamel junction

Initial apical pressure

Rapid, small clockwise counter-clockwise rotational movements

90° rotation buccal toward midline

Stubbie forceps

Figure 4.2   Extraction of a maxillary canine tooth.

4) **Final Check.** Confirm the tooth number and location with radiograph.
5) **Local Anaesthetic.** Infiltration of the buccal vestibule will provide sufficient anaesthesia for the maxillary buccal soft tissue and periodontal ligament. Localised palatal infiltration is required to anaesthetise the palatal gingiva.
6) **Positioning.** Lie the patient flat in the dental chair, with the maxillary canine at the same vertical height as the surgeon's elbow. Stand on the side of the patient that corresponds with the hand dominance of the surgeon. For example, a right-handed practitioner standing on the right side of the patient increases biomechanical advantage when removing the tooth.
7) **Elevation.** Apply the straight elevator to the mesial and distal areas of the periodontal ligament. Using a wheel-and-axle motion, gently expand the periodontal ligament until a small amount of mobility is noted in the tooth. Take care to elevate between tooth and bone only, and not against adjacent teeth. The thumb and finger of the nondominant hand should be used to support the alveolus of the tooth being extracted, to guide the application of force to the tooth socket only, and to prevent instrument slippage.
8) **Delivery.** Apply the beaks of the stubbie forceps on to the cementoenamel junction of the tooth. Initially, use apical pressure to slide the beaks as deep on to the root as possible. Employ a rapid clockwise–counterclockwise rotational movement to continue tearing the periodontal ligament. Finally, rotate the crown 90° to deliver the crown and root.
9) **Assessment.** Assess the tooth root to ensure it has been removed complete. Flush the socket with saline to remove any surgical debris. Examine the socket for bleeding, alveolar bone fracture, or soft tissue trauma, and manage as appropriate.

4.3   Maxillary Premolars

1) **Difficulty Assessment.** Maxillary first premolars always have two roots: buccal and palatal. Maxillary second premolars may have either two separate roots or two roots fused together (Figure 4.3). Root configuration should be assessed radiographically; this should be correlated clinically, as maxillary premolars are commonly found to be rotated slightly, which can affect the vectors of extraction. As with all multirooted teeth, complex root configurations warrant surgical extraction.
2) **Obtain Consent.** General risks apply for maxillary premolar teeth.
3) **Basic Equipment Required.** Upper universal forceps can be used for all maxillary premolars. The curved handle of the instrument allows for ideal placement of the beaks without interfering with the lower arch. A straight elevator should be available to expand the periodontal ligament prior to forceps placement.
4) **Final Check.** Confirm the tooth number and location with radiograph.
5) **Local Anaesthetic.** Infiltration of the buccal vestibule will provide sufficient anaesthesia for the maxillary buccal soft tissue and periodontal ligament. Localised palatal infiltration is required to anaesthetise the palatal gingiva.
6) **Positioning.** Lie the patient flat in the dental chair, with the maxillary molars at the same vertical height as the surgeon's elbow. Stand on the side of the patient that corresponds with the hand dominance of the surgeon. For example, a right-handed practitioner standing on the right side of the patient increases biomechanical advantage when removing the tooth.
7) **Elevation.** Apply a straight elevator to the mesiobuccal aspect of the periodontal ligament. Using a wheel-and-axle motion, gently push the tooth in a distal direction. Care should be taken to not use excessive force during this movement, as root fractures commonly occur at this stage. Only a

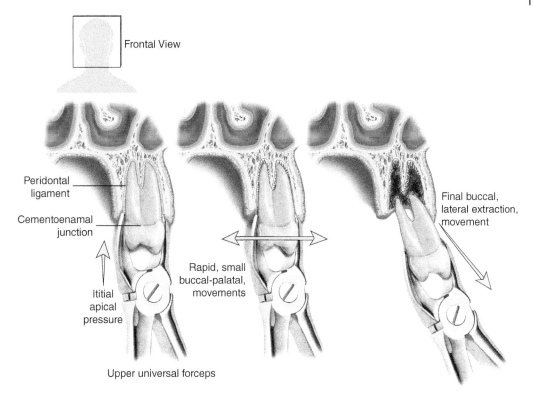

Figure 4.3 Extraction of a maxillary premolar tooth.

slight amount of tooth mobilisation is required before progressing to tooth delivery. The thumb and finger of the nondominant hand should be used to support the alveolus of the tooth being extracted, to guide the application of force to the tooth socket only, and to prevent instrument slippage.

8) **Delivery.** Apply the beaks of the upper universal forceps on to the cementoenamel junction of the tooth. Initially, use apical pressure to slide the beaks as deep on to the roots as possible. Employ rapid, small, buccopalatal movements to expand the socket. Rotation of upper premolars is not recommended as this goes against the strongest axis of the tooth and may cause root fracture. Excessive palatal tilting is also not recommended as this will cause palatal root fracture, necessitating surgical extraction. Complete the extraction with a final buccal movement, to deliver the tooth laterally.

9) **Assessment.** Assess the tooth root to ensure it has been removed complete. Flush the socket with saline to remove any surgical debris. Examine the socket for bleeding, alveolar bone fracture, or soft tissue trauma, and manage as appropriate.

4.4 Maxillary First and Second Molars

1) **Difficulty Assessment.** The multirooted nature of maxillary molars warrants early consideration of a surgical extraction approach over simple extraction (Figure 4.4). In younger individuals (less than 40 years of age), a simple extraction is likely to be successful; in older individuals, where other maxillary teeth in the posterior region have been removed already, attempting a simple extraction can be difficult, and fraught with complications. Radiographically, assessment

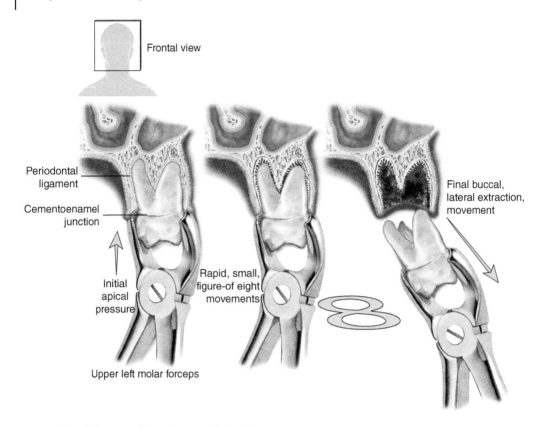

Frontal view

Periodontal ligament

Cementoenamel junction

Initial apical pressure

Rapid, small, figure-of eight movements

Final buccal, lateral extraction, movement

Upper left molar forceps

Figure 4.4 Extraction of a maxillary molar tooth.

of the root configuration will give the first indication that surgical extraction may be indicated, due to splaying of roots. The surgeon must also assess for pneumatisation of the sinus from extractions of adjacent teeth; this indicates that the bone between the tooth and maxillary sinus is very thin and is likely to fracture during extraction, with subsequent oroantral communication. Worse, displacement of the tooth or roots into the maxillary sinus cavity can occur.

2) **Obtain Consent.** In addition to the generic extraction risks, patients must be informed of the risk of oroantral communication or displacement of tooth roots into the sinus. Both outcomes may require secondary surgery or referral to a specialist oral and maxillofacial surgeon and can have a significant effect on the prosthetic rehabilitation of the newly edentulous site. If the maxillary second molar is being removed, patients must be warned of the risk of tuberosity fracture.

3) **Basic Equipment Required.** Upper left or right molar forceps are designed specifically for the typical root configuration of upper molars; that is, the beaks of the forceps are designed to adapt around two buccal roots and one palatal root. A straight elevator should be kept available at all times. Occasionally, other elevators may be required to remove fractured root fragments.

4) **Final Check.** Confirm the tooth number and location with radiograph.

5) **Positioning.** Lie the patient flat in the dental chair, with the maxillary premolars at the same vertical height as the surgeon's elbow. Stand on the side of the patient that corresponds with the hand dominance of the surgeon. For example, a right-handed practitioner standing on the right side of the patient increases biomechanical advantage when removing the tooth.

6) **Elevation.** Use a straight elevator at the mesiobuccal line angle of the tooth. Use a wheel-and-axle motion subgingivally, to elevate between tooth and bone, and break the periodontal ligament. Only 1–2 mm of crown movement is required after elevation. Excessive elevation can cause crown or root fracture and should be avoided, as this may necessitate a switch to a surgical approach. The thumb and finger of the nondominant hand should be used to support the alveolus of the tooth being extracted, to guide the application of force to the tooth socket only, and to prevent instrument slippage.

7) **Delivery.** Apply the beaks of the upper molar forceps on to the cementoenamel junction of the tooth. Initially, use apical pressure to slide the beaks as deep on to the roots as possible. Employ rapid, small, figure-of-eight movements to expand the buccal bone. As upper molars may have three or four roots, care should be taken to avoid excessive movement in one direction only, until the tooth complex is mobile enough to deliver complete using a final buccal movement.

8) **Assessment.** Assess the tooth root to ensure it has been removed complete. Flush the socket with saline to remove any surgical debris. Examine the socket for bleeding, alveolar bone fracture, or soft tissue trauma, and manage as appropriate. If an oroantral communication is noted, this requires immediate management (see Chapter 6).

4.5 Mandibular Incisors

1) **Difficulty Assessment.** Extraction of mandibular incisors is made simple by their single-rooted nature, relative lack of major root curvatures, and ease of access (Figure 4.5). Lower anterior teeth are a common subsite for advanced periodontal disease, due to the accumulation of calculus in this area; this can be the most common indication for extractions in the anterior mandible. Anterior mandibular bone can be unwieldy, however, and root fracture is a likely result if excessive force is placed on the tooth along an incorrect vector. Sharp luxators should be used with extreme care, as excessive force can cause slippage into the floor of the mouth, where many vital structures may be damaged, necessitating advanced surgical repair.

2) **Obtain Consent.** General risks of dental extraction apply for mandibular incisors. Any prosthetic rehabilitation plan for anterior teeth should be specifically included in the consent process for any tooth in the smile line.

3) **Basic Equipment Required.** A lower universal or lower root forceps can be used for mandibular central and lateral incisors, depending on the diameter of the tooth root. A straight elevator may be used to expand the periodontal ligament prior to extraction, but this should be approached with extreme care to avoid slippage.

4) **Final Check.** Confirm the tooth number and location with radiograph.

5) **Local Anaesthetic.** Infiltration of the buccal vestibule will provide sufficient anaesthesia for the maxillary buccal soft tissue and periodontal ligament. Localised lingual infiltration may be required to anaesthetise the lingual gingiva. For multiple anterior mandibular extractions, bilateral mental nerve blocks can be used to anaesthetise the entire anterior sextant from canine to canine, as local anaesthetic can diffuse through the mental foramen and cause profound retrograde anaesthesia.

6) **Positioning.** Sit the patient upright, with the mandibular teeth at the same vertical height as the surgeon's elbow. Stand on the side of the patient that corresponds with the hand dominance of the surgeon. For example, a right-handed practitioner standing on the right side of the patient increases biomechanical advantage when removing the tooth, compared to standing on the opposite side.

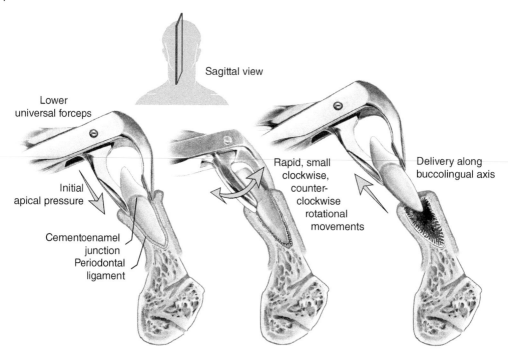

Figure 4.5 Extraction of a mandibular incisor tooth.

7) **Elevation.** Apply the straight elevator to the mesial and distal areas of the periodontal ligament. Using a wheel-and-axle motion, gently expand the periodontal ligament until a small
   amount of mobility is noted in the tooth. Take care to elevate between tooth and bone only, and
   not against adjacent teeth. As the cross-section of lower anterior roots is more ovoid in the buccolingual direction and narrower in the mesiodistal direction, excessive mesiodistal elevation
   of the tooth may cause root fracture. The thumb and finger of the nondominant hand should be
   used to support the alveolus of the tooth being extracted, to guide the application of force to the
   tooth socket only, and to prevent instrument slippage.
8) **Delivery.** Apply the beaks of the forceps on to the cementoenamel junction of the tooth. Initially,
   use apical pressure to slide the beaks as deep on to the roots as possible. Mandibular anterior soft
   tissues are extremely delicate, so care must be taken not to impinge them in the forceps, as large
   soft tissue tears may result. Since the strongest cross-sectional axis of the tooth is buccolingual,
   elevation and subsequent delivery of the tooth must occur along this axis to avoid root fracture.
9) **Assessment.** Assess the tooth root to ensure it has been removed complete. Flush the socket
   with saline to remove any surgical debris. Examine the socket for bleeding, alveolar bone fracture, or soft tissue trauma, and manage as appropriate.

4.6 Mandibular Canines and Premolars

1) **Difficulty Assessment.** As with maxillary canines, the extraction of mandibular canines can
   be deceptively difficult, due to their large root surface, thick buccal and lingual alveolar bone,
   and reduced periodontal ligament space (Figure 4.6). More often than not, a surgical approach
   is necessitated when little crown remains, as there is no purchase from which to grasp the tooth

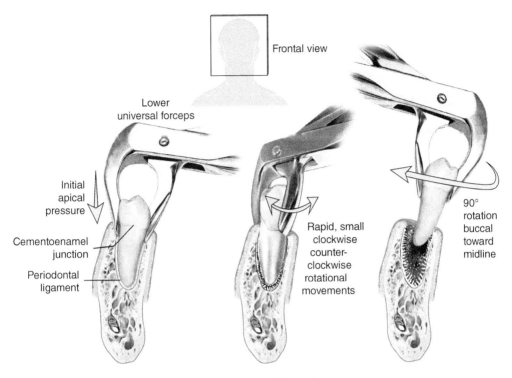

Figure 4.6 Extraction of a mandibular canine or premolar tooth.

root and apply sufficient force to deliver it from the mouth. Buccal alveolar plate fractures are very common with mandibular canine extraction and should be accounted for in difficulty assessment. Mandibular premolar teeth are similar to mandibular canines in terms of difficulty, and can be approached in the same fashion.

2) **Obtain Consent.** In addition to the general risks of dental extraction, patients should be specifically informed of the risk of buccal alveolar fracture, as this can be common with removal of canines, and can affect future prosthetic rehabilitation.

3) **Basic Equipment Required.** Lower universal forceps are well suited for removing lower canine teeth and premolars. A wide, straight elevator should be available to expand the periodontal ligament prior to forceps placement.

4) **Final Check.** Confirm the tooth number and location with radiograph.

5) **Local Anaesthetic.** Infiltration of the buccal vestibule and lingual gingiva should provide sufficient anaesthesia for the mandibular buccal soft tissue and periodontal ligament of the canine. For premolar teeth, an inferior alveolar nerve block, a lingual nerve block, and buccal infiltration are all required to produce sufficient anaesthesia for extraction.

6) **Positioning.** Sit the patient upright, with the mandibular teeth at the same vertical height as the surgeon's elbow. Stand on the side of the patient where the teeth are being extracted, regardless of surgeon hand dominance. For example, lower left canines and premolars should be approached from the left side, whilst lower right canines and premolars should be approached from the right.

7) **Elevation.** Apply the straight elevator to the mesial and distal areas of the periodontal ligament. Using a wheel-and-axle motion, gently expand the periodontal ligament until a small amount of mobility is noted in the tooth. Take care to elevate between tooth and bone only, and not against adjacent teeth. The thumb and finger of the nondominant hand should be used to

support the alveolus of the tooth being extracted, to guide the application of force to the tooth socket only, and to prevent instrument slippage.

8) **Delivery.** Apply the beaks of the lower universal forceps on to the cementoenamel junction of the tooth. Initially, use apical pressure to slide the beaks as deep on to the root as possible. As the roots of lower canines and premolars are conical and usually straight, a rapid clockwise–counterclockwise rotational movement can be used to continue tearing the periodontal ligament. Finally, rotate the crown 90° to deliver the crown and root together.

9) **Assessment.** Assess the tooth root to ensure it has been removed complete. Flush the socket with saline to remove any surgical debris. Examine the socket for bleeding, alveolar bone fracture, or soft tissue trauma, and manage as appropriate.

4.7 Mandibular Molars

1) **Difficulty Assessment.** Mandibular molars can be difficult to extract using simple techniques alone (Figure 4.7). Appropriate engagement of a molar tooth with forceps is entirely dependent on the integrity of the tooth crown; deep subgingival caries are a sound indication for an early surgical approach. Molar teeth have at least two roots, but can have up to four. Roots are often divergent or may have a bridge of cancellous bone passing between them, locking the tooth in place and preventing removal. Rarely, they can be fused together, necessitating surgical sectioning and delivery of individual roots. This is further complicated by the dense and unforgiving nature of bone in the

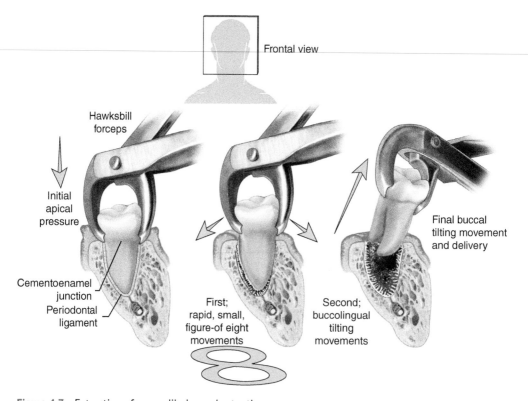

Figure 4.7 Extraction of a mandibular molar tooth.

posterior mandible, the potential presence of lingual tori, and the limited access to posterior areas by buccal soft tissues. The most common problem encountered during extraction of mandibular teeth is a low root tip fracture, which can be very difficult to salvage. The proximity of mandibular molar roots to the inferior alveolar nerve canal should be assessed radiographically, as any attempts to extract root tips without due care may cause displacement into the inferior alveolar nerve canal.

2) **Obtain Consent.** General risks of dental extraction apply for mandibular molars. Additionally, the patient should be informed of the risk of temporary or permanent paraesthesia following extraction.

3) **Basic Equipment Required.** Two forceps options are available for removal of lower molar teeth. **Hawksbill forceps** are designed to engage a large portion of the circumference of the cementoenamel junction, like other forceps, allowing maximum rotational forces to be applied favourably. They are useful when the crown of a molar tooth is intact, but tend to fail and cause root fracture if there is crown compromise. **Cowhorn forceps** engage the furcation of the tooth only; whilst this increases the likelihood of crown fracture, this fracture tends to propagate between the roots and effectively sections the mesial and distal portions of the tooth. These forceps also allow for subgingival engagement in situations where there is extensive crown decay. A wide, straight elevator should be available to expand the periodontal ligament prior to forceps placement.

4) **Final Check.** Confirm the tooth number and location with radiograph.

5) **Local Anaesthetic.** Inferior alveolar nerve block, lingual nerve block, and buccal infiltration are all required to produce sufficient anaesthesia for extraction.

6) **Positioning.** Sit the patient upright, with the mandibular teeth at the same vertical height as the surgeon's elbow. For the right-handed surgeon, removal of right mandibular molars is best approached standing behind the patient, to maximise mechanical advantage, whilst left mandibular molars are best removed standing on the patient's left. The opposite holds for the left-handed surgeon: stand behind the patient when extracting left mandibular molars and on the patient's right when extracting right mandibular molars.

7) **Elevation.** Apply the straight elevator to the mesial and distal areas of the periodontal ligament. Using a wheel-and-axle motion, gently expand the periodontal ligament until a small amount of mobility is noted in the tooth. Take care to elevate between tooth and bone only, and not against adjacent teeth. The thumb and finger of the nondominant hand should be used to support the alveolus of the tooth being extracted, to guide the application of force to the tooth socket only, and to prevent instrument slippage.

8) **Delivery.** When using hawksbill forceps, apply the instrument to the cementeoenamel junction of the tooth, in a position that maximises contact between the tooth and the beaks. Employ rapid, small, figure-of-eight movements to expand the buccal bone, followed by buccolingual tilting movements to mobilise the tooth. Once the tooth complex is mobile enough to deliver complete, use a final buccal tilting movement. With cowhorn forceps, again apply the instrument to the cementeoenamel junction, engaging the furcation between the mesial and distal root structures. Use a crushing force initially, to wedge the cowhorn beaks into the furcation of the tooth causing the tooth to dislodge and to become easy to deliver using a buccal tilting movement. Rather than delivering the tooth, this crushing force may instead cause a favourable fracture of the crown between the mesial and distal roots; this allows each half of the tooth – each now a separate crown–root complex – to be delivered separately using lower universal forceps, as if it were a single-rooted tooth.

9) **Assessment.** Assess the tooth root to ensure it has been removed complete. Flush the socket with saline to remove any surgical debris. Examine the socket for bleeding, alveolar bone fracture, or soft tissue trauma, and manage as appropriate.

5

Surgical Extraction Techniques

In certain clinical situations, use of simple extraction instruments is insufficient to deliver an entire tooth and its roots in a safe and uncomplicated manner. Attempts to remove such teeth using simple methods only can be time-consuming and inefficient, and can expose the patient to undue risk or discomfort. In these situations, a surgical approach to tooth extraction is indicated. This chapter introduces the basic techniques of surgical extraction.

Historically, the terms 'intra-alveolar' and 'transalveolar' were used to differentiate extractions that could be performed with forceps alone from extractions that required advanced surgical techniques such as flap raising, bone removal, and tooth sectioning. Over time, these terms have become less representative of extraction difficulty or techniques required. This is largely due to the development of atraumatic extraction techniques for dental implant placement, where extractions are performed within the intra-alveolar structures, but use the same advanced surgical techniques of traditional trans-alveolar extraction. This terminology has thus now largely been replaced with 'simple extraction' and 'surgical extraction', respectively, as this better represents the kinds of pre-surgical planning required for tooth removal.

The distinction between 'simple' and 'surgical' dental extractions is still somewhat difficult to define. From a technical perspective, surgery by nature involves the manipulation of tissues of the body; as such, extraction of teeth with forceps and luxators is still within the realm of dentoalveolar 'surgery'. Furthermore, use of the descriptive term 'simple' has been misconstrued to be synonymous with 'low in difficulty' – this, in fact, is not necessarily the case. Finally, it is not uncommon that a dental extraction procedure that is planned as a 'simple' extraction needs to be converted to a 'surgical' extraction due to intraoperative complications or unexpected difficulties that inhibit completion of the procedure.

In pragmatic terms, a 'surgical extraction' implies the use of additional surgical methods to successfully complete dental extraction, including soft tissue manipulation and flap raising, removal of bone, and sectioning of teeth using a rotary instrument (Table 5.1). Situations where a surgical extraction is indicated include (Table 5.2):

- **Preoperatively**, where, in the difficulty assessment stage, it is determined that use of luxators and dental extraction forceps alone will be insufficient to safely and completely remove the tooth.
- **Intraoperatively**, where:
  - either the whole tooth or part of the tooth is unable to be removed with simple methods alone ('failed extraction');

Principles of Dentoalveolar Extractions, First Edition. Seth Delpachitra, Anton Sklavos and Ricky Kumar.
© 2021 John Wiley & Sons Ltd. Published 2021 by John Wiley & Sons Ltd.
Companion website: www.wiley.com/go/delpachitradentoalveolarextractions

Table 5.1   General steps in surgical extraction.

1) Obtain appropriate anaesthesia.
2) Raise mucoperiosteal flap.
3) Remove bone.
4) Section tooth.
5) Create point of elevation, if required.
6) Elevate roots.
7) Debride socket.
8) Achieve haemostasis and suture surgical site.

Table 5.2   Situations where surgical extraction methods may be required.

History of difficult extraction
Large body habitus
History of failed extraction
Structural issues with the tooth from caries or previous root canal therapy
Complex roots
Bulbous roots
Hypercementosis
Clinical suspicion of ankylosis or dense alveolar bone

- excessive damage is occurring to the surrounding hard and soft tissues due to the level of force required to remove the tooth using simple extraction instruments; or
- the time taken to remove the tooth is greater than expected or the patient is experiencing significant discomfort.

5.1   General Principles of Surgical Extraction

A number of key principles must be followed when planning a surgical extraction:

1) **Appreciate the Anatomy of Maxillofacial Neurovascular Structures.** The clinical decision to manipulate the hard and soft tissues of the oral cavity can significantly increase the risk associated with an oral procedure. During 'simple' extractions, there are no vital structures that are likely to be encountered in the routine removal of a tooth from the oral cavity. When soft tissues are cut or elevated, however, care must be taken to reduce the risk of stretching or transecting neurovascular bundles in the vicinity of the surgical site. Arterial vessels abound and have a highly unpredictable course within the face, and failure to account for their location, or to stay in the appropriate tissue plane, can lead to significant blood loss. Using surgical burs to drill bone without a clear estimation of its structural integrity or that of its surrounding structures can lead to unexpected nerve injury, oroantral communication, or intraoperative bony fracture.
2) **Understand the Principles of Soft Tissue Flap Design.** The key one being access: the success or failure of a procedure, and its difficulty, can be entirely dependent on the soft tissue flap used. The specific design of the flap is of less importance than the principles on which it is based – principles that support sufficient access, minimal soft tissue handling and inadvertent trauma, and neat, tension-free apposition of the flap at the conclusion of surgical extraction.

3) **Use the Correct Burs and Instruments.** The traditional dental handpieces and instruments are not sufficient to perform surgical extraction. Purpose-designed instruments are required for safe and careful soft tissue manipulation and dissection, as outlined in Chapter 3. Similarly, traditional high- and slow-speed handpieces attached to a pneumatic dental setup are not suitable for surgical procedures and may cause serious injury to the patient.

4) **Recognise the Indication for Surgical Extraction.** In order to perform successful surgical extraction, it may be prudent to ask: 'Why could this tooth not be removed using simple extraction techniques?' The answer to this question will always provide the framework through which a surgical approach can be planned. For example, awareness that a tooth cannot be removed due to impaction in bone prepares the practitioner to use a soft tissue flap and bone removal techniques to access it for extraction. Similarly, noting preoperatively the presence of splayed roots without a clear vector for extraction informs the practitioner that sectioning of the roots may be required.

5) **Manage the Outcomes of Surgical Extraction.** Surgery, by its nature, implies an increased manipulation of the tissues in order to achieve the desired outcome. Manipulation of soft tissues through flap raising at the start of a procedure should be followed by adequate approximation of the same tissues at the end of the procedure. Failure to do so can result in persistent haemorrhage from the surgical site, large wound dehiscences, infections, and a poor postoperative result.

5.2 Practical Aspects of Surgical Extraction

Mucoperiosteal flaps involve elevation of the 'full thickness' of oral tissues abutting the maxilla and mandible. All tissues (mucosa, submucosa, muscle, periosteum) are raised in a single layer, following the cleavage plane formed between bone and periosteum. This form of soft tissue flap, whilst not the only type, is the most common, safe, and versatile method of accessing the hard tissues for completion of surgical extractions.

A well-designed soft tissue flap can provide excellent access for immediate bone removal and tooth sectioning during dentoalveolar surgical procedures. However, a poorly designed one – not following proper principles – can lead to increased difficulty of dental extraction in the short term and, more importantly, significant damage to the periodontium and gingiva over the long term. Flap necrosis and gingival recession can be a costly and difficult problem to correct as a result of poor soft tissue management.

1) **Use as Large an Incision as Necessary.** The key principle of flap design is to provide access to the relevant underlying structures. In situations where it may be reasonably expected that more access will be required, the flap should be designed to allow for this.

2) **Provide a Broad Soft Tissue 'Base' to Maintain Tissue Vascularity to the Tip of the Flap and Ensure the Width of the Flap is Twice as Long as Its Height.** Flaps with a narrower pedicle may undergo avascular necrosis at the crestal areas, resulting in large periodontal defects.

3) **Place the Incision Over Sound Bone Without Bony Prominences.** Bony prominences create tension at wound edges, which may promote wound breakdown and dehiscence.

4) **Avoid Placing the Incision Directly Over an Area that May Be a Bony Defect By the End of the Procedure.** It is not uncommon that a large defect will exist at the end of bone removal and dental extraction. Flaps heal poorly if the wound edges are not against a stable bony surface, due to increased tension at the suture site causing localised ischaemia.

5) **Avoid Incisions that Transect the Crestal Gingiva on the Buccal Convexities of the Teeth.** The gingiva is thinnest and under most tension at the midpoint of the buccal gingiva. Incisions in this area that are not carefully repaired can lead to long-term periodontal dehiscence, which may require future periodontal surgery to normalise the clinical crown length. If a relieving incision is to be used that transects the gingiva, it should be closer to the interdental papillae, as these areas are much less likely to dehisce due to increased tissue bulk.

6) **Avoid Incising Near Neurovascular Structures.** The mental foramen, inferior orbital foramen, lingual nerve, incisive nerve, and greater palatine artery are all susceptible to iatrogenic injury if their position is not factored into the design of a soft tissue flap. Transection of these structures will result in irreversible anaesthesia, paraesthesia, or dysaesthesia for the patient.

7) **Use Sharp, Clean, and Precise Incisions to Enable Apposition of the Soft Tissues During Closure.** Jagged or poorly defined edges result in a less than ideal closure, which can lead to wound breakdown and future localised periodontal disease.

8) **Follow the Cleavage Planes of the Soft Tissues.** A mucoperiosteal flap is most robust when all layers (mucosa, submucosa, muscle, and periosteum) are raised together. Failure to maintain a subperiosteal plane predisposes the flap to avascularity or tearing.

5.3 Common Soft Tissue Flaps for Dental Extraction

A **crestal or envelope approach** involves an incision made in the sulcus of the gingiva surrounding teeth and elevation of a mucoperiosteal flap from the bony alveolar crest away from the tooth (Figure 5.1). The gingival papillae are incised between the teeth at the interproximal col to provide as long and broad a pedicle as possible, and to maintain the blood supply to both the buccal and the lingual sides of the transected papillary tip. The envelope approach provides excellent access to the crestal alveolar bone and periodontal structures, but access is limited to the stretch of the

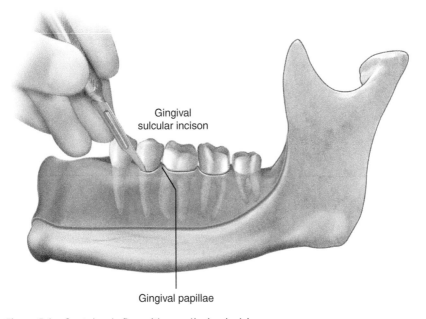

Gingival sulcular incison

Gingival papillae

Figure 5.1   Crestal-only flap with no relieving incision.

keratinised gingival tissue. If deeper apical areas of the tooth or bone require access, use of a crestal incision alone can lead to unfavourable tearing of the flap, which will require careful apposition.

Raising of a crestal flap commences with the sharp gingival sulcular incision along the region of keratinised gingiva that is to be elevated from the bone. A fine scalpel, such as an #11 or #15 blade, is best suited for this task.

Once the sulcus is incised, the pointed end of a periosteal elevator should first be used to free the gingival papillae away from the interdental areas. This area is usually the most tethered, and freeing of the papillae early helps to prevent flap tearing along the remainder of the gingival margin. Once the papillae have been freed, the remainder of the flap can be elevated from the bone, taking care to remain in the subperiosteal plane at all times.

After the surgical procedure is completed, apposition of the flap should be undertaken with interdental mattress sutures to correctly apposition the gingival papillae.

Relieving incisions are apical extensions of a crestal flap that can be used to improve bony exposure through transection of the keratinised gingival margin. Relieving incisions may be placed at the mesial end of the incision (Figure 5.2), at the distal end, or at both the mesial and the distal ends (Figure 5.3). The decision as to where a relieving incision should be made depends upon the area and amount of access required and the surrounding neurovascular structures, with an emphasis on reducing damage to the periodontal tissues as much as possible. Relieving incisions cannot be used alone, as they do not provide access to the required underlying tissues without an associated crestal component.

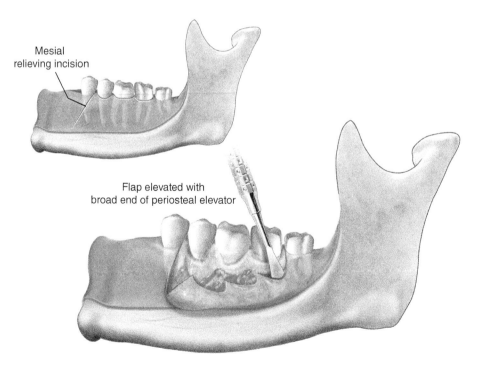

Mesial
relieving incision

Flap elevated with
broad end of periosteal elevator

Figure 5.2   Two-sided flap, consisting of a crestal flap with mesial relieving incision.

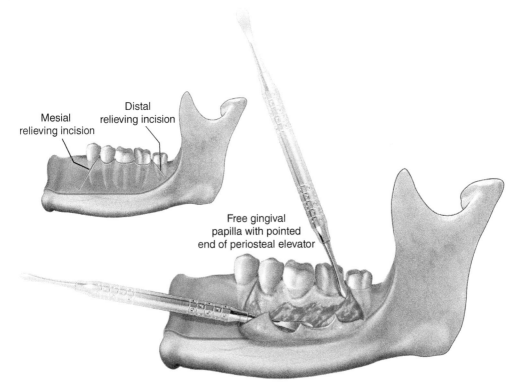

Mesial relieving incision

Distal relieving incision

Free gingival papilla with pointed end of periosteal elevator

Figure 5.3 Three-sided flap, consisting of a crestal flap with mesial and distal relieving incisions.

The decision to use a relieving incision may be made after a crestal flap has already been raised, but ideally this should be decided upon beforehand. In either situation, the technique is the same, although it is more difficult if the crestal flap has already been raised, as the tissues are harder to put under tension. Once an appropriate retractor has been used to place tension on the area to be incised, a sharp blade should be used to create a relieving incision through the full thickness of the mucoperiosteal flap. The relieving incision should start at the crestal interdental gingiva, including the adjacent gingival papilla, and end once the free mucosa is reached. Care should be taken to avoid neurovascular structures, such as the mental or inferior orbital nerves, when the relieving incision is in the vicinity of these anatomic areas. Once the flaps have been appropriately incised, they can be gently elevated using the broad end of the periosteal elevator.

When the surgical procedure is completed, large relieving incisions should be reattached using a mattress suture through the included papilla of the flap. It is not essential to obtain primary closure of the incision through the free mucosa; in fact, this opening can be used as a port for surgical drainage.

In situations where a tooth is impacted within the soft and hard tissue, away from the crowns of the erupted dentition, a **vestibular incision** can be used to spare iatrogenic damage to the periodontium and gingiva of that dentition (Figure 5.4). A common example is the buccally erupted upper canine tooth, which can lie as high as the piriform rim. Vestibular incisions are confined to the free mucosa only, and as such, any flaps raised are extremely versatile and offer excellent access to underlying structures.

Vestibular incisions should only be used if the tooth marked for extraction is sufficiently distant from the keratinised gingiva, as the incision requires an adequate 'cuff' of mucosa on either side to allow for closure, without putting tension on the gingiva, which can cause recession.

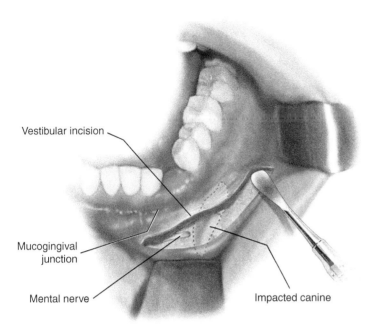

Figure 5.4 Vestibular incision used to approach an impacted canine.

To perform a vestibular incision, first the mucosa must be placed under tension. The incision should be at least 3 mm away from the mucogingival junction, and may be parallel to this line or slightly convex from it. The first incision should be made through and perpendicular to the mucosa. Once the mucosa is incised, a second pass should be made with the scalpel down through submucosa and periosteum to bone. The flap can then be gently elevated with a broad periosteal elevator to expose the underlying bone and impacted tooth.

When the procedure is completed, the vestibular incision can be opposed using simple interrupted sutures or a continuous-suture technique.

5.4 Bone Removal

Once a tooth and the overlying alveolar bone is exposed, bone removal may be required in order to:

1) Eliminate any bony impaction of the crown of an impacted tooth.
2) Remove bone around bulbous roots, where the diameter of the root is too great and impedes delivery of a tooth root from the socket.
3) Create an application point whereby an elevator can be used to wedge between tooth root and bone to facilitate elevation of the root.

Precision is the key factor in performing successful bone removal. Appropriately planned bone removal ensures that the periodontal space between tooth and bone is maintained, to provide a precise application point for a dental elevator. Careful removal of bone around adjacent tooth roots and nerves prevents iatrogenic damage to these structures, which helps to prevent postsurgical complications.

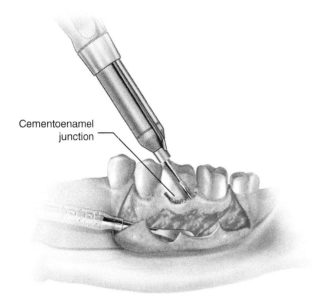

Cementoenamel
junction

Figure 5.5 Buccal bone gutter to facilitate removal of a lower molar.

Planning where bone is to be removed depends on the desired outcome of the removal. In most cases, bone removal is undertaken to create a straight and open path of delivery for a tooth or tooth root (Figure 5.5). As such, the bone removed should be predominantly at the cementoenamel junction of the tooth, as wide as possible without damaging adjacent teeth, and only as apical as is required to bypass the thickest part of the tooth, all whilst enabling a point of access for instrumentation.

With the advent of immediate dental rehabilitation with endosseous implants, emphasis should be placed on the preservation of as much alveolar bone as possible. Adequate alveolar bone height and width can be maintained through techniques that, where possible, favour tooth sectioning over bone removal, in order to remove teeth.

Using an appropriate retractor, the soft tissues must be kept away from the site where bone is to be removed. A round or fissure bur attached to a surgical handpiece should be used to gently remove the bone around the desired area, starting from where the crown is visible. In nearly all cases, exposure of the entire crown to the cementoenamel junction is considered sufficient bone removal, although this can vary depending on the complexity of the case, and more or less may be required to obtain the desired outcome. Care must be taken not to drill into the tooth itself, as this can lead to loss of anatomy or difficulty in maintaining an application point, whilst at the same time creating a point of weakness that may lead to crown fracture. Irrigation should be used throughout bone removal to prevent thermal osteonecrosis, and surgical suction must be applied liberally to collect any irrigant and debris from the site.

5.5 Tooth Sectioning

Once a tooth's crown is sufficiently exposed, and bone removal has provided sufficient exposure of the tooth roots and space for extraction, tooth sectioning should be performed, if required. Generally, tooth sectioning is utilised in three situations: crown removal, to create space to

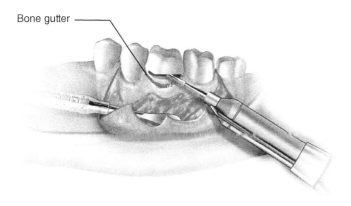

Bone gutter

Figure 5.6   Decoronation of a tooth.

facilitate root removal; sectioning between multirooted teeth; and sectioning axially along a single-rooted tooth.

Decoronation (separation of a crown from its roots) can assist in creating a path of exit when elevating the root in situations where the crown is impacted (Figure 5.6). Even when the crown is not impacted, removal can still be a useful technique to visualise the root anatomy of a multirooted tooth and provide additional access for further bone removal and sectioning. To decoronate a tooth, the cementoenamel junction should first be exposed from under any hard or soft tissue. A straight bur must be held perpendicularly to the tooth. The tooth can then be sectioned through the entire depth of the crown, taking care not to traverse through the crown into surrounding structures. The section should be completed using an elevator to remove the crown.

Sectioning between roots can be used for multirooted teeth, where each root may have a different vector of extraction (Figure 5.7). Sectioning between roots allows for extraction of each root individually, and reduces the risk of excessive force on alveolar bone. It is easiest to perform (although this is not absolutely necessary) after decoronation of a tooth, as pulp and root anatomy is easier to identify, and access to the interradicular areas of the root system is far simpler. An understanding of the root anatomy and recognition of the variations in the preoperative assessment is essential when undertaking root sectioning. If roots are not sectioned according to tooth anatomy, undesirable fractures of root tips can occur, leading to a much more complex and lengthy procedure.

Sectioning within a single root is usually reserved for canine teeth, where a wide single-rooted tooth with a large periodontal ligament area is resistant to removal and the surrounding alveolar bone is thick and unforgiving (Figure 5.8). In order to preserve alveolar bone, the tooth may be sectioned axially through the pulp chamber. This allows each half of the root to be luxated into the resultant space and elevated separately. Sectioning in such a fashion is an advanced skill, but when appropriately utilised, it significantly improves the prognosis of the area for future prosthetic rehabilitation.

5.6   Cleanup and Closure

Once a tooth has been extracted, the socket should be examined for any tooth remnants, debris, or iatrogenic damage to the periodontal bone or soft tissues. This involves gently irrigating the socket

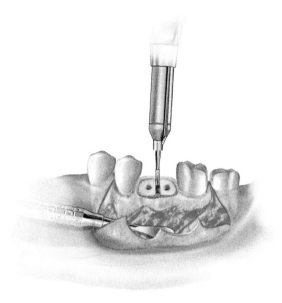

Figure 5.7 Sectioning between roots.

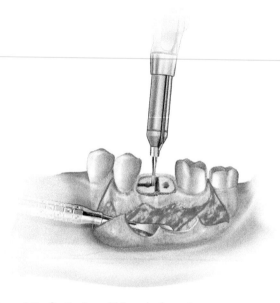

Figure 5.8 Sectioning within a single root.

with 5–10 ml of normal saline; if any periodontal plaque or calculus is noted on the adjacent teeth, these areas should be gently curetted to reduce the risk of postoperative infection.

The socket and surrounding areas should be checked for any frank bleeding that may need to be addressed. A transient ooze is expected following extraction, but prolonged bleeding lasting more than five minutes requires active management. If there is bleeding from alveolar bone after an uncomplicated extraction, the precise source must first be discovered. A resorbable gelatin- or cellulose-based dressing can then be packed against the area.

The final step in surgical extraction is closure of the socket. Using interrupted sutures, any soft tissue flaps must be repositioned to their original locations, with a particular emphasis on restoring the periodontal contour of the alveolus. The socket itself can be left slightly open to facilitate surgical drainage from the site, which can reduce postoperative pain and swelling.

6

Intraoperative Complications

Intraoperative complications are an unavoidable risk of undertaking surgery. Whilst often unpredictable, a comprehensive preoperative assessment, good surgical insight, and adequate planning can lead to minimisation of risk and timely management of the pending complication to avoid future problems. This chapter reviews the common intraoperative complications encountered during simple extraction, and how they can be predicted and subsequently managed.

All forms of surgery require the use of traumatic instruments, in a controlled manner, in order to produce energy against the bodily tissues. This controlled tissue trauma minimises the damage done to the adjacent tissues during surgery, delivering a planned and predictable postoperative result. With the use of such instruments, however, comes the risk that trauma may instead occur in an *uncontrolled* manner. It is through this mechanism that most intraoperative complications occur.

Whilst safe practice and insight can minimise the risk of such complications, it is inevitable that the dentoalveolar surgeon will encounter each of those listed in this chapter at least once during their career. In such situations, the minimisation of harm to the patient is the goal of immediate management.

6.1 Lip Burns and Lacerations

The mobile lips and cheeks are the largest obstacle between the surgeon and the surgical site, and add an additional layer of difficulty compared with other forms of surgery. Lip lacerations usually occur as a result of inadvertent contact with the sharp metal instruments on their entry and exit from the oral surgical site. Lip burns are largely the result of inadequate retraction of the tissues when using a surgical handpiece. Both are significant complications, as they may cause long-term, visible external scarring or stricturing, in extreme cases requiring advanced facial plastic surgery.

If a lip burn or laceration occurs during a procedure, this needs to be evaluated immediately, before continuing with the planned surgery. The area should be examined for any obvious bleeding from the tissues and managed with firm pressure initially. All trauma must be clearly documented and described. Most importantly, the tissues involved – mucosa, vermillion, or skin – should be identified, as this will have a major impact on the prognosis of the patient.

Principles of Dentoalveolar Extractions, First Edition. Seth Delpachitra, Anton Sklavos and Ricky Kumar.
© 2021 John Wiley & Sons Ltd. Published 2021 by John Wiley & Sons Ltd.
Companion website: www.wiley.com/go/delpachitradentoalveolarextractions

Minor mucosal lacerations or burns generally carry a good prognosis, given the ability of the mucosa to heal without scarring. Minor burns may be managed conservatively, with observation five days post-event to assess healing. Superficial mucosal lacerations that are amenable to closure may be sutured using a fast resorbable suture, to reapproximate edges and promote healing.

Larger mucosal burns or burns and lacerations involving the vermillion border or external facial skin require tertiary referral to a specialist oral and maxillofacial surgeon. Referral must be made promptly, so that any required treatment can be provided without delay.

When this complication is encountered, communication with the patient is key. Damage to the lips should be clearly listed and discussed in the preoperative setting. Post-injury, patients must be informed regarding the nature of the incident, tissues involved, likely prognosis, and disposition for advanced surgical care, if needed.

6.2 Damage to Adjacent Teeth or Restorations

Elevator instruments are designed to be wedged between a tooth being extracted and the surrounding alveolar bone. Use of elevators therefore applies force in two directions: against the tooth being extracted, but also against the bone.

Improper use of elevators may see them being placed between the tooth being extracted and an adjacent tooth, exposing the latter to extraction forces. This can lead to either luxation of the entire adjacent tooth or, more likely, damage to the structural integrity of that tooth's crown or restorations. Situations where this is likely are usually predictable during the preoperative assessment, through examination of the radiograph for the periodontal integrity of the adjacent teeth or for the presence of large restorations or crowns (Figure 6.1).

Luxation of adjacent teeth is a difficult problem to manage. As soon as there is any clinical suspicion that an adjacent tooth has been mobilised, the procedure should be stopped, and the area examined to ensure there is no associated dentoalveolar complex fracture. Once an adjacent tooth has been mobilised, elevator instruments become unsuitable for continuation of the extraction;

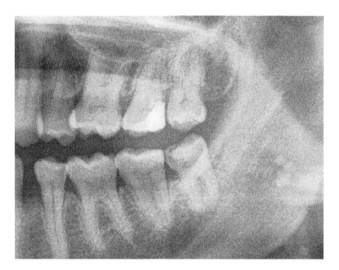

Figure 6.1   Upper second molar showing heavy restoration, putting it at high risk of iatrogenic injury if care is not taken during removal of the upper third molar.

either forceps only should be utilised or surgical methods must be adopted. Once the tooth marked for extraction has been removed, standard trauma management of a luxated or avulsed tooth should be applied.

Where the adjacent teeth have been previously restored, this restoration is susceptible to dislodgement or breakage, as it does not carry the structural strength of a native, unrestored tooth. Dislodgement of large restorations creates an additional intraoperative problem that must be addressed. Any broken restoration material or fractured enamel should be removed from the surgical site, as this may pose an airway risk or elicit a foreign-body reaction if inadvertently pushed into the soft tissues. The extraction must be completed carefully, without the use of elevators near the broken tooth. The patient must be informed of the incident, and of the need for temporisation of the previously restored area. This should occur immediately, with a future definitive restorative plan arranged after the immediate postoperative period.

6.3 Mandible Fracture

If exerted inappropriately on mandibular teeth, the forces of extraction may lead to fracture of the mandible. This serious complication is more often than not the result of a failure to recognise the reason why a tooth may not be mobilising, and the use of excessive force in a direction of weakness of the mandibular bone. It commonly occurs in patients with atrophic mandibles or short mandibular body height, or where attempts are made to remove an impacted tooth without use of surgical techniques by a novice practitioner. Fractures may also be encountered in patients with osteoporosis or abnormal pathologic processes in the area, such as cysts or tumours.

Mandible fracture may be suspected if there is a loud 'crack' heard, associated with increasing pain, and loss of continuity of the mandibular teeth with stepping or diastemas. Gingival lacerations may be evident, with surrounding haematomas.

If clinically suspected, mandible fracture must be ruled out with radiograph prior to proceeding with extraction. The radiographic appearance of a radiolucent, irregular line passing obliquely or perpendicularly to the mandible bone is diagnostic of fracture. If evident, attempts to remove the tooth should cease immediately. This complication requires emergency treatment under general anaesthetic by a specialist oral and maxillofacial surgeon, and the patient should be referred to the nearest tertiary referral hospital for inpatient management.

6.4 Tooth Aspiration or Ingestion

Loss of a tooth into the oropharynx is a medical emergency and should be treated as such until proven otherwise. In the worst-case scenario, a tooth can enter the tracheobronchial tree, causing airway obstruction and cardiorespiratory arrest. More likely, however, is that the patient's gag reflex is activated, triggering either a swallow – causing the tooth to be ingested into the gastrointestinal tract – or a vomit expelling the contents of the stomach and elevating the tooth out of the upper airway.

If a tooth is lost into the oropharynx, the patient should be managed according to basic life support protocols. If there are signs of impending respiratory obstruction, the patient requires immediate ambulance transfer to the nearest hospital for bronchoscopy and removal of foreign body. Their airway must be secured, and high-flow oxygen applied via mask. If the patient is unresponsive or not breathing, cardiopulmonary resuscitation should be commenced until the arrival of paramedic personnel.

If the patient is clinically stable, transfer to a local emergency department is still required, to confirm the location of the lost tooth with a chest x-ray; this is imperative, as patients may still be clinically stable even if tooth fragments are present in the tracheobronchial tree. If the tooth has been swallowed and is in the stomach, it will most likely pass through the alimentary system and excreted in faeces.

6.5 Instrument Fracture

Instrument fractures only occur when there is a pre-existing defect in the instrument being used or when fine instruments are used for a purpose for which they are not designed. This is most commonly seen with the use of a fine periotome to simultaneously disrupt the periodontal ligament of a tooth and elevate a large tooth. Periotomes have a small, sharp end that is an efficient cutting instrument, but is not designed to withstand rotational force along its axis.

If instrument fracture occurs, it is imperative that the fractured components be removed carefully. Fractured instrument components may act as a nidus of infection or elicit a foreign body granulomatous reaction that can culminate in acute osteomyelitis of the bone. A surgical approach may be necessitated to remove the fractured segments, possibly requiring deeper surgical exploration of the surgical site once the tooth has been extracted.

6.6 Intraoperative Bleeding

During or after extraction of a tooth, bleeding is a common complication. Whilst it generally stops spontaneously, failure to manage intraoperative bleeding may lead to life-threatening postoperative bleeding, which can result in haematoma or ecchymosis, and require blood transfusion or hospitalisation.

Intraoperative bleeding may result from trauma to the soft tissues, causing laceration of blood vessels, or from bone trauma, resulting in bleeding from nutrient canals or central bone vessels. It can be exacerbated by the presence of inflammation or infection, due to the vasodilatory effect of inflammatory mediators. A number of medical conditions can contribute to increased bleeding risk, and these require specific assessment and management prior to any surgical procedures.

Intraoperative bleeding during dental extractions that is unexpected must be stabilised prior to patient discharge. Whilst a number of methods and materials are available for haemostasis, use of the principles of pressure, packing, and patience is the first (and often only) method required to obtain sufficient haemostasis. In nearly all cases, the best course of action is to remove the tooth first, prior to application of haemostatic measures; the exception is in situations where bleeding is profuse and significant, where the tooth may be utilised as a well-adapted pressure dressing (e.g. where a high-flow arteriovenous malformation is encountered).

Immediate pressure to the area using a gauze bite pack for approximately 5–10 minutes provides enough time for the surgeon to prepare for additional haemostatic agents, if required (Table 6.1), and for the tissues and vessels to progress through vasospasm and platelet plug formation. A reduced flow of haemorrhage allows for a thorough examination of the surgical site in a systematic manner, commencing with the soft tissues surrounding the extraction site, through to all bony windows of the tooth socket, and finally to the apex of the socket. Occasionally, a single bleeding point is identifiable; more commonly, the intraoperative haemorrhage is a general ooze from all of the tissues. If a single bleeding point is found, specific local measures may be used to control the

Table 6.1 Haemostatic agents that may be used to assist with control of bleeding after dental extraction.

Local anaesthetic infiltration
Suturing
Gauze pressure ± impregnation
Cellulose
Gelatin foam
Thrombin
Fibrin
Tranexamic acid mouthwash
Calcium alginate
Bone wax

bleeding in the area. Bone wax is a useful tool for this purpose, where intrabony vessels require plugging.

If generalised oozing is present, a simple method of haemostasis is to pack the socket with an absorbable haemostatic agent of choice and then place a retention suture over it. Additional pressure with haemostatic gauze soaked in 0.2% tranexamic acid solution or 1 : 100000 adrenaline for 30 minutes increases the haemostatic effect.

Patients with significant intraoperative bleeding that cannot be controlled may require urgent referral to the closest emergency department for further investigation and haemorrhage control. This should be organised promptly in discussion with the local oral and maxillofacial surgery service.

6.7 Oroantral Communication

An oroantral communication is a direct hole between the oral cavity and the maxillary sinus. The most common cause is extraction of a lone-standing posterior maxillary tooth, with an associated fracture of the thin alveolar bone that separates the two cavities. This usually occurs in the context of lone-standing solitary upper first molars or high-impacted upper third molars; however, any tooth that has roots anatomically close to the sinus cavity may be at risk. Occasionally, oroantral communications can be associated with displacement of a tooth root or fragment into the maxillary sinus.

The likelihood of oroantral communication from an upper first molar may be precisely determined preoperatively on the panoramic radiograph, based on the relationship of the sinus floor to the root of the tooth. If the floor of the antrum lies below more than one-quarter of the distance between the apex and the cementoenamel junction, the risk of oroantral communication is considered high.

The surgeon may only be alerted to the presence of an oroantral communication after tooth extraction has been completed. Large oroantral communications will be visible on examination of the socket; irrigation with normal saline will produce the sensation of water trickling down the back of the patient's nose, as the fluid passes directly into the maxillary sinus and on to the nasal cavity. Smaller ones can be identified by asking the patient to Valsalva whilst holding the nares shut; airflow or bubbles in the socket may be appreciable. At no stage should the socket be instrumented, as this has the potential to either create or worsen an oroantral communication.

Oroantral communications may close spontaneously when the defect has a width of less than 5 mm. Defects over this size are unlikely to close spontaneously and require surgical repair. This should occur promptly, as, if untreated, 50% of patients will develop acute bacterial sinusitis after 48 hours. Partial oroantral communications, where the bony sinus floor is breached but the maxillary sinus membrane is intact, generally do not require surgical intervention and will heal uneventfully.

If an oroantral communication is not detected intraoperatively, patients may present within one to two weeks postoperatively with symptoms of regurgitation of liquids between the nose and mouth, air passage between the two cavities, altered vocal resonance, or symptoms suggestive of sinusitis.

Repair of oroantral communication and removal of displaced root fragments from the maxillary sinus is an advanced surgical skill that is performed by specialist oral and maxillofacial surgeons. The patient should be appropriately informed of this complication, and a semi-urgent outpatient referral to a specialist service is necessary. Given the propensity for these patients to develop acute bacterial sinusitis, a course of preoperative empirical oral antibiotics with sinus coverage should be prescribed, along with saline nasal sprays for lavage.

6.8 Dentoalveolar Fracture

Lone-standing teeth that have been under repetitive, heavy cycles of load are more likely to be ankylosed to the underlying bone. Clinically, these teeth will often respond differently to standard approaches to elevation and delivery using dental instruments. In situations where a tooth is ankylosed, dentoalveolar fracture is the unintended consequence of tooth extraction.

Dentoalveolar fractures may range in presentation from a small piece of alveolus attached to the root surface to large dentoalveolar fragments where there is separation of a large complex of bone with attached teeth from the maxilla or mandible (Figure 6.2). In larger fragments, there may be involvement of surrounding structures, which may need to be addressed. For example, large dentoalveolar segment fractures of the posterior maxilla are a frequent cause of later oroantral communication.

The surgeon should be suspicious of dentoalveolar fracture in cases where abnormally high amounts of force are required to mobilise a tooth, or if there is abnormal or unexpected movement of the adjacent teeth or under the soft tissues. A large 'crack' may or may not be associated with creation of a dentoalveolar fracture. Patients may experience pain associated with the fracture if it extends past the area of local anaesthesia.

If the presence of a small buccal alveolar bone fracture is noted, the surgeon's aim should be to remove the tooth safely, preserving the gingival soft tissues. If the fractured segment only covers the root surface of the tooth being extracted, it is appropriate to use a periosteal elevator to gently separate the fractured bone from the gingiva, then remove the tooth and fractured segment as a single piece. Any soft tissue trauma should be addressed and sutured, where necessary.

If the fractured segment extends to the root surfaces of adjacent teeth, the surgeon should attempt to preserve as much soft tissue attachment to the piece of bone as possible, and to separate the tooth being extracted from the ankylosed bone segment. This requires gentle and careful luxation; if the tooth cannot be successfully released from the bony segment, the segment will have to be sacrificed. This comes at the cost of future periodontal problems for the adjacent teeth and should be avoided where possible. If the bone segment can be salvaged, a tight approximation of

Small Dentoalveolar Fracture

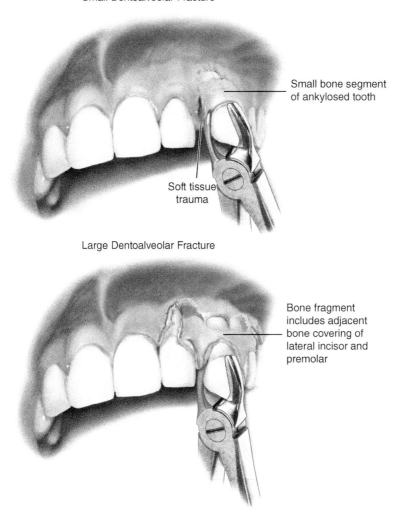

Small bone segment
of ankylosed tooth

Soft tissue
trauma

Large Dentoalveolar Fracture

Bone fragment
includes adjacent
bone covering of
lateral incisor and
premolar

Figure 6.2   Small and large dentoalveolar fractures.

the soft tissues is essential in order to reposition this fractured segment, which is now essentially biologically identical to a free bone graft, and is susceptible to future necrosis and sequestration.

When the fractured segment is large and other teeth are attached to the fractured complex, repositioning and rigid splinting of the segment is the priority, to allow for bony healing and salvage of as many teeth as possible. Whilst fractures of this nature can appear disastrous, appropriate repositioning and splinting using traumatology principles carries an excellent prognosis. The tooth extraction procedure should be delayed as long as is safely possible until bone healing is complete, at approximately four weeks post-repositioning. A surgical approach is then necessary, in order to reduce the amount of force required for future attempts at tooth extraction.

7

Third Molar Surgery

This chapter introduces the practice of third molar surgery, including classification systems, difficulty assessment, indications, and surgical approach.

Extraction of third molar ('wisdom') teeth is a unique aspect of dentoalveolar surgery, and carries additional challenges in treatment planning and approach. The decision to remove wisdom teeth is not as straightforward as that to remove other teeth with pathology; in fact, in some centres worldwide, the prophylactic removal of asymptomatic, pathology-free third molars is advocated, for a number of reasons. This removal is not without risks and complications, and remains an area of controversy.

The main predictive factor underlying third molar impaction appears to be inadequate space between the distal part of the second molar and the ascending ramus. This can be influenced by a relatively small jaw, relatively large teeth, and the presence of crowding in the dentition, as well as the age of the patient. However, even amongst expert dentists and oral and maxillofacial surgeons, the ability to predict future impaction based upon these findings on panoramic radiography is poor, particularly in younger populations.

Third molar teeth are complex and difficult to remove, for a number of reasons:

- The indications for their removal are different than those for general tooth extraction.
- Third molars that require removal nearly always have some form of hard or soft tissue impaction, which needs to be addressed when planning for removal; that is, wisdom tooth removal is almost exclusively a surgical extraction, as opposed to a simple one.
- Mandibular third molars may be in close proximity to the inferior alveolar nerve and the lingual nerve.
- Maxillary third molars are closely related to the maxillary sinus, maxillary tuberosity, and related vascular structures.
- Postoperative complications relating to infection can be worse than with other teeth, given the proximity of the third molar to surrounding deep neck spaces.

7.1 Treatment Planning of Impacted Third Molars

The list of indications for third molar extraction is extensive: extraction may be indicated for symptoms or pathology associated with the wisdom teeth themselves, their effects on the wider dentition, or as part of a wider comprehensive dental or medical treatment plan (Tables 7.1 and 7.2).

Principles of Dentoalveolar Extractions, First Edition. Seth Delpachitra, Anton Sklavos and Ricky Kumar.
© 2021 John Wiley & Sons Ltd. Published 2021 by John Wiley & Sons Ltd.
Companion website: www.wiley.com/go/delpachitradentoalveolarextractions

Table 7.1 Indications for third molar extraction as per the National Institute for Health and Care Excellence (NICE) and the American Association of Oral and Maxillofacial Surgeons (AAOMS).

NICE guidelines (UK)	AAOMS indications (USA)
Recurrent history of infection (including pericoronitis)	Pain
	Carious tooth
Unrestorable caries	Pericoronitis
Nontreatable pulpal and/or periapical pathology	Facilitation of the management of or limitation of progression of periodontal disease
Cellulitis, abscess, and osteomyelitis	Nontreatable pulpal or periapical lesion
Periodontal disease	Acute and/or chronic infection (e.g. cellulitis, abscess)
Prophylactic removal in the presence of specific medical and surgical conditions	Ectopic position (malposition, supraeruption, traumatic occlusion)
Facilitation of restorative treatment (including provision of prosthesis)	Abnormalities of tooth size or shape precluding normal function
Internal and/or external resorption of tooth or adjacent teeth	Facilitation of prosthetic rehabilitation
Pain directly related to the third molar	Facilitation of orthodontic tooth movement and promotion of stability of the dental occlusion
Tooth in the line of fracture of the mandible	Tooth in the line of fracture complicating fracture management
Fracture of the tooth	Tooth involved in surgical treatment of associated cysts and tumours
Disease of the dental follicle (including cyst and tumour)	Tooth interfering with orthognathic and/or reconstructive surgery
Tooth or teeth impeding orthognathic or reconstructive surgery	Preventive or prophylactic removal, when indicated, for patients with medical or surgical conditions or treatments (e.g. organ transplants, alloplastic implants, bisphosphonate therapy, chemotherapy, radiation therapy)
Teeth involved in the field of tumour resection	
Tooth suitable for use as a donor for transplantation	Clinical findings of pulp exposure by dental caries
	Clinical findings of fractured tooth or teeth
Orthodontic treatment (e.g. maxillary retraction)	Impacted tooth
	Internal or external resorption of tooth or adjacent teeth
	Patient's informed refusal of nonsurgical treatment options
	Anatomic position causing potential damage to adjacent teeth
	Use of the third molar as a donor tooth for tooth transplant
	Tooth impeding the normal eruption of an adjacent tooth
	Resorption of an adjacent tooth
	Pathology associated with the tooth follicle

Table 7.2 Contraindications for third molar extraction.

Extremes of age

Complex medical history, which can lead to significant postoperative morbidity (e.g. a history of radiotherapy to the region)

Situations where there is a high risk of intraoperative complications requiring tertiary-level services or general anaesthetic (e.g. high risk of mandible fracture)

Situations where an acute problem impacts access or local anaesthesia (e.g. acute odontogenic infection with trismus)

Table 7.3 Treatment options for third molar teeth based upon presence of symptoms and presence of pathology.

	Symptoms	No symptoms
Pathology	1) REMOVE	1) REMOVE
No pathology	1) REMOVE	1) MONITOR
	2) MONITOR	2) REMOVE
	3) OPERCULECTOMY	

The presence of third molar teeth is most commonly alerted to the patient by routine panoramic radiography performed by the general dentist, or by the onset of symptoms related to eruption or impaction. Generally, third molar teeth can be classified into four categories based on the presence of symptoms and the presence of periodontal pathology (Table 7.3). Symptoms can include pain, recurrent facial infections, and pericoronitis with food impaction. Pathology includes the presence of clinical signs of periodontal disease.

1) **Symptomatic With Clinical Signs of Disease.** Patients with symptoms and clinical signs of disease will largely benefit from removal of the third molar. In most cases, complete removal of the tooth, rather than conservative or minor surgical methods (e.g. operculectomy), is required to remove the associated pathology.
2) **Symptomatic Without Clinical Signs of Disease.** In this category, patients present with symptoms of pain or swelling, without evidence of developing impaction. Observation with symptom control is an appropriate means of managing these cases until their clinical prognosis becomes clearer with time. If symptom control methods are inadequate to provide sufficient patient comfort, extraction may be indicated. Similarly, these teeth may be removed alongside other third molars as part of a whole-of-mouth treatment plan.
3) **Asymptomatic With Clinical Signs of Disease.** This group of impacted third molars is detected on clinical examination in patients who have never exhibited symptoms but are noted to have periodontal pocketing, dental caries, or the presence of an operculum. Prophylactic removal of these teeth is recommended, to prevent periodontal defects to the adjacent second molar.
4) **Asymptomatic Without Clinical Signs of Disease.** The prophylactic removal of asymptomatic, disease-free third molars in this category has been suggested, in order to prevent the need for future third molar extractions in older age groups with greater case difficulty and surgical risk. However, there is insufficient literature to support this practice. Management of teeth in this category should be determined on a case-by-case basis, considering the individual circumstances that may determine patient prognosis.

7.2 Difficulty Assessment and Preoperative Workup

The major challenge in planning wisdom tooth extraction is the broad diversity of anatomic impactions, clinical presentations, and indications, and the extensive number of factors which can influence the difficulty of an individual case. The difficulty assessment phase of treatment planning is the most crucial deciding factor in terms of the success versus failure of a procedure, and in determining whether the case should be referred to a specialist oral and maxillofacial surgeon. Great

Table 7.4 Local and general factors that increase the difficulty of third molar removal.

Local factors	Depth of impaction and type
	Root formation
	Proximity to inferior alveolar canal
	Caries or periodontal disease
	Mouth opening
	Gag reflex
General factors	Patient psychological factors
	Age
	Sex
	Ethnicity
	Patient weight

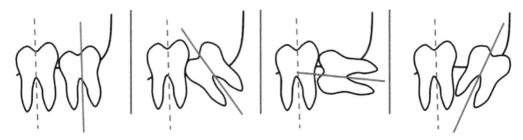

Figure 7.1 Winter's classification of third molars. From left to right: vertical impaction, mesioangular impaction, horizontal impaction, distoangular impaction. *Source:* Freire, B.B., Nascimento, E.H.L., Vasconcelos, K. de F., Freitas, D.Q., & Haiter-Neto, F. (2019). Radiologic assessment of mandibular third molars: an ex vivo comparative study of panoramic radiography, extraoral bitewing radiography, and cone beam computed tomography. *Oral Surgery, Oral Medicine, Oral Pathology and Oral Radiology*, 128(2), 166–175. © 2019 Elsevier.

care must be taken when deciding which wisdom teeth fall within the scope of the practitioner, as failed extractions can lead to significant morbidity for the patient, and to serious medicolegal concerns.

A comprehensive difficulty assessment involves the assessment of local and systemic factors, as well as indications and contraindications, for each individual scenario (Table 7.4).

Whilst a number of methods have been described for the classification of wisdom tooth impaction, there is poor correlation between any of them and the overall operative difficulty; this requires a much more comprehensive assessment of the patient. However, these classification systems can still be utilised as a method of communication between practitioners and patients, and can help to guide the surgical approach.

Winter's classification is based upon the orientation of the third molar tooth's axis relative to the adjacent second molar (Figure 7.1). Mesioangular third molars have an axis that is tilted in a mesial direction towards the second molar. Distoangular third molars have an axis tilted in a distal direction away from the second molar. Vertical third molars have an axis parallel to the second molar. Horizontal third molars have an axis perpendicular to the second molar.

On the basis of this classification, the general surgical approach to each type of impaction will be outlined later in this chapter. Keep in mind that the surgical principles described in Chapter 6 must always be adhered to with regards to soft tissue access, judicious bone removal, and sectioning of the tooth, where appropriate, in order to successfully complete the extraction.

7.3   Radiographic Assessment of Inferior Alveolar Nerve Risk

A **panoramic radiograph** is the minimum requirement for radiographic assessment of third molars. There are two reasons for this. First, a whole-of-mouth approach is required when determining the role of third molar extractions as part of an overall treatment plan. Second, the relationships of the third molars to their surrounding structures is best represented on a panoramic radiograph rather than on intraoral radiographs, which may be difficult to obtain in the most posterior areas of the oral cavity.

The assessment of a panoramic radiographic begins with a systematic and thorough examination of the whole radiograph for other incidental pathologic findings. Next, attention is paid to the wisdom teeth themselves, noting the size, location, type of impaction, root formation, presence of associated pathology (e.g. odontogenic cysts or tumours, periodontal pathology, or dental caries), and relationship to surrounding structures.

Of particular importance to mandibular third molars is the relationship of the roots to the inferior alveolar nerve. Damage to the inferior alveolar nerve can cause temporary or permanent anaesthesia, paraesthesia, or dysaesthesia, all of which may be extremely unpleasant for the patient and contribute to long-term morbidity. As such, avoidance of nerve injury during wisdom tooth extraction is of critical importance. There are seven radiographic signs that may be associated with injury to the inferior alveolar nerve, three of them (in bold) significantly so (Figure 7.2):

1) **Darkening of the root**
2) Deflection of the root
3) Narrowing of the root
4) Bifid root apex
5) **Interruption of the 'white line' of the canal**
6) **Diversion of the canal**
7) Narrowing of the canal

Importantly, inferior alveolar nerve injury may still occur even in the absence of these signs. However, the presence of any of them warrants additional radiographic investigation with CBCT and referral to a specialist oral and maxillofacial surgeon for further management.

7.4   Surgical Approach to Third Molars

In any approach to third molar extractions, the basic equipment required, final check, and local anaesthetic techniques are all largely the same as for other mandibular molar surgical extractions. For maxillary third molars, buccal and palatal infiltration anaesthetic is required to produce sufficient anaesthesia for extraction. For mandibular third molars, inferior alveolar nerve block, lingual nerve block, and buccal infiltration are required.

7.4.1   Maxillary Third Molars

7.4.1.1   Erupted

Despite full crown eruption, maxillary third molars are usually indicated for extraction due to buccal or lingual positioning of the tooth, as a result of inadequate space. Maxillary third molars have a variable crown size and root configuration, which must be factored into the method of removal. Generally speaking, the approach to erupted maxillary third molars should mimic that to removal of a maxillary second molar; in situations where surgical extraction may be indicated (e.g. unfavourable root configuration), the principles of surgical extraction should be applied.

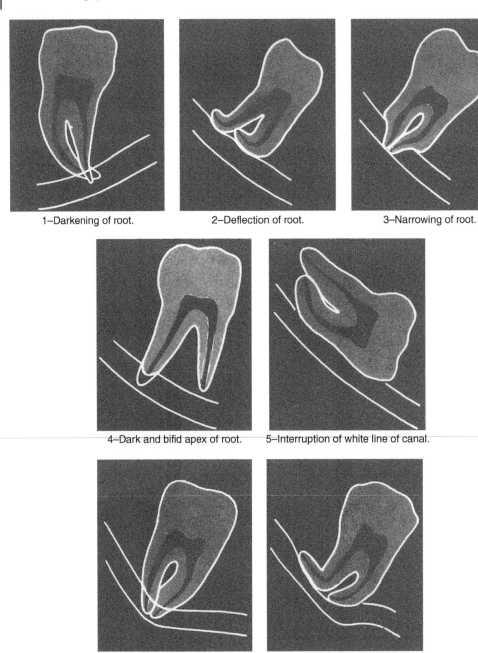

1–Darkening of root.   2–Deflection of root.   3–Narrowing of root.

4–Dark and bifid apex of root.   5–Interruption of white line of canal.

6–Diversion of canal.   7–Narrowing of canal.

Figure 7.2 Radiographic signs that may be associated with an increased risk of damage to the inferior alveolar nerve during third molar extraction. *Source:* J.P. Rood, B.A.A. Nooraldeen Shehab, The radiological prediction of inferior alveolar nerve injury during third molar surgery, *British Journal of Oral and Maxillofacial Surgery*, Volume 28, Issue 1, 1990, Pages 20–25. https://doi.org/10.1016/0266-4356(90)90005-6. Reprinted by permission from Elsevier.

7.4.1.2 Unerupted/Partially Erupted

The surgical approach to teeth in this category begins with adequate soft tissue exposure. A crestal incision with distal relieving arm, or alternatively an East Grinstead slash, is used to expose the crown of the tooth. It is rare to require bone removal, even in partly developed maxillary third molars, as the maxillary bone is soft and usually thin around the tooth crown. If a small amount of bone removal is required, it should be sufficient to provide an application point on the mesiobuccal aspect between crown and alveolus. A curved elevator (e.g. a Warwick-James or Cryer) is used to elevate the tooth in a distobuccal direction and deliver the crown and roots. As with all surgical extractions, the socket should be irrigated and checked for debris and alveolar integrity, and the flap repositioned and sutured.

7.4.2 Mandibular Third Molars

The approach will vary significantly depending on the type and depth of impaction. This section provides a basic approach to each type of impaction, but it must be acknowledged that due to the great variability in presentations of mandibular third molar teeth, a number of different approaches are valid in each case; the choice should be based upon clinician preference and experience.

7.4.2.1 Mesioangular

1) **Soft Tissue Access.** Raise an envelope flap from the absolute distal of the second molar, extending to the mid-buccal gingival margin of the first molar. A small distal relieving incision, including any partly erupted component of the third molar, lengthens this incision approximately 5 mm along the external alveolar ridge. If it is predicted that extensive bone removal is required, a mesial reliving incision or triangular flap should be considered. Elevate the flap gently using a periosteal elevator to expose the underlying crown and alveolus. Once the flap has been mobilised, retract and protect it with an appropriate retractor (e.g. a Minnesota retractor).
2) **Bone Removal.** Identify the bony margin between the alveolus and the crown of the third molar. Gently drill a buccal 'gutter' along the mesiobuccal to distobuccal surfaces of the crown, deep enough to expose the cementoenamel junction of the tooth. Sufficient bone should be removed as far distal as possible along the crown of the third molar at the ascending ramus, as this is the main point of bony impaction.
3) **Tooth Sectioning.** Perform an axial section, as far along the length of the root as possible, to separate the mesial and distal halves of the tooth. If the tooth has two roots, mesial and distal, the aim of this section is to separate them at the furcation. In single-rooted third molars, the aim is to remove as much of the distal part of the crown as possible, in order to create space for elevation. If axial sectioning is technically difficult, decoronation may be used as a first step to remove the crown and provide access to the root complex for further sectioning. Each time part of the tooth is sectioned with a drill, an elevator is used to separate and mobilise the tooth segments.
4) **Delivery.** Generally speaking, elevate the most distal part of the crown, with or without its attached distal root, first. Once this has been removed, access to the mesial portion of the tooth is easier, and this portion can be elevated into the resulting space. If there are root fragments remaining in the socket, remove these last.
5) **Cleanup and Closure.** Assess the tooth root to ensure it has been removed complete. Flush the socket with saline to remove any surgical debris. Examine the socket for bleeding, alveolar bone fracture, or soft tissue trauma, and manage as appropriate. Finally, reposition the flap, using a suture at the distal of the 7 to reoppose this section first, followed by additional sutures on the relieving incisions as required (Figure 7.3).

7.4.2.2 Distoangular/Vertical

1) **Soft Tissue Access.** Raise an envelope flap from the distal of the second molar, extending to the papilla between the first and second molars. A large distal relieving incision approximately

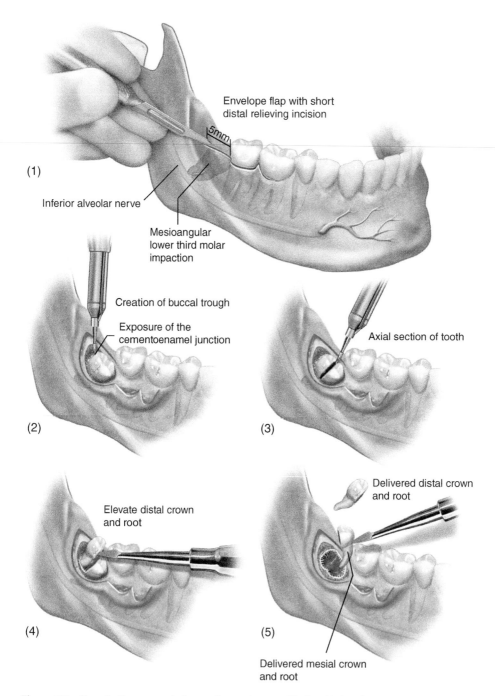

(1)

Envelope flap with short
distal relieving incision

5mm

Inferior alveolar nerve

Mesioangular
lower third molar
impaction

(2)

Creation of buccal trough

Exposure of the
cementoenamel junction

(3)

Axial section of tooth

(4)

Elevate distal crown
and root

(5)

Delivered distal crown
and root

Delivered mesial crown
and root

Figure 7.3 Steps in the removal of a mesioangular mandibular third molar.

5–10 mm along the external alveolar ridge should be added to the envelope, including any partly erupted component of the third molar, to allow for predominant exposure of the distal crown and ascending ramus. Elevate the flap using a periosteal elevator, exposing the crown and alveolus. Retract and protect the flap with an appropriate retractor.

2) **Bone Removal.** Identify the bony margin between the alveolus and the crown of the third molar. Gently drill a buccal 'gutter' along the buccal to distal surfaces of the crown, deep enough to expose the cementoenamel junction of the tooth. Most of the bone removal during a distoangular tooth extraction is on the furthest distal part of the crown, which is often difficult to access due to the ascending ramus; a large amount of bone removal is thus required to ensure success.

3) **Tooth Sectioning.** Axial sectioning of distoangular or vertical teeth is difficult in the context of limited access and given the length of the surgical bur. As such, removal of the distal two-thirds of the crown is the first step in tooth sectioning. Do not remove whole crown at this point; leaving the mesial portion provides an application point for elevation, and maintaining some crown assists in providing anatomic reference points relative to the root.

4) **Delivery.** Complete the sectioning and remove the distal portion of the crown with a straight elevator. Once this has been done, elevate the remaining crown–root complex into the space, using a straight elevator wedged between the mesial edge of the third molar and the alveolus. If the tooth is multirooted, the roots may require individual sectioning prior to elevation and removal.

5) **Cleanup and Closure.** Assess the tooth root to ensure it has been removed complete. Flush the socket with saline to remove any surgical debris. Examine the socket for bleeding, alveolar bone fracture, or soft tissue trauma, and manage as appropriate. Finally, reposition the flap, using a suture at the distal of the 7 to reoppose this section first, followed by additional sutures on the relieving incisions as required (Figure 7.4).

Note that whilst vertically impacted mandibular third molars can sometimes be extracted using simple methods, this is often not the case, due to the limited access to the posterior mandible obtained using conventional extraction instruments. As such, whilst vertical impactions may appear technically simple on panoramic radiograph, the clinician must always be prepared to employ surgical techniques to successfully complete the extraction.

7.4.2.3 Horizontal

1) **Soft Tissue Access.** Horizontally impacted mandibular third molars require a large access, as the amount of bone removal needed to expose the crown of the tooth is significant. An envelope flap, extending to the mid-buccal area of the first molar, with an approximately 5–10 mm distal relieving incision along the external alveolar ridge, affords excellent exposure of the crown and alveolar bone.

2) **Bone Removal.** Use a fissure or round bur to remove alveolar bone from the superior surface of the tooth, until the cementoenamel junction has been exposed. Once this is done, continue bone removal along the buccal surface of the tooth, creating a deep buccal gutter that extends along the entire buccal-facing surface of the crown. Such extensive bone removal is necessary to provide space for luxation, as the third molar is often wedged firmly against the root of the second molar.

3) **Tooth Sectioning.** Almost always, decoronation at the cementoenamel junction is the best first step towards approaching a horizontally impacted third molar. Removal of the crown in one or more pieces affords visualisation and access to the root complex, which can then be addressed secondarily. However, it is important to note that the inferior alveolar nerve may lie directly underneath the crown of a horizontally impacted third molar; extreme care must thus be taken not to section completely through the tooth with the bur, as iatrogenic injury to this nerve is likely. Instead, use a bur to section through three-quarters of the total width of the tooth, and complete the section atraumatically with a large elevator (a Coupland elevator is useful for this purpose).

4) **Delivery.** Deliver the crown of the tooth in one or more pieces using a small elevator. Once the crown has been removed, examine the remaining root complex. Further sectioning between the roots may be required to deliver each root individually.

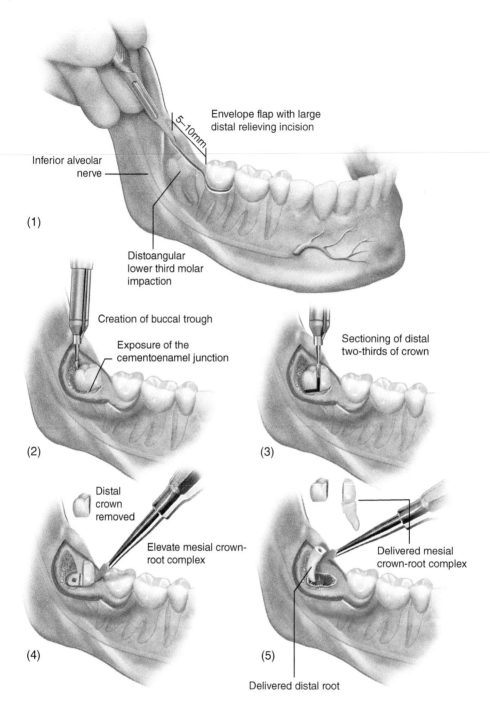

Envelope flap with large distal relieving incision

5–10mm

Inferior alveolar nerve

(1)

Distoangular lower third molar impaction

Creation of buccal trough

Exposure of the cementoenamel junction

(2)

Sectioning of distal two-thirds of crown

(3)

Distal crown removed

Elevate mesial crown-root complex

(4)

Delivered mesial crown-root complex

(5)

Delivered distal root

Figure 7.4 Steps in the removal of a distoangular mandibular third molar.

5) **Cleanup and Closure.** Assess the tooth root to ensure it has been removed complete. Flush the socket with saline to remove any surgical debris. Examine the socket for bleeding, alveolar bone fracture, or soft tissue trauma, and manage as appropriate. Finally, reposition the flap, using a suture at the distal of the 7 to reoppose this section first, followed by additional sutures on the relieving incisions as required (Figure 7.5).

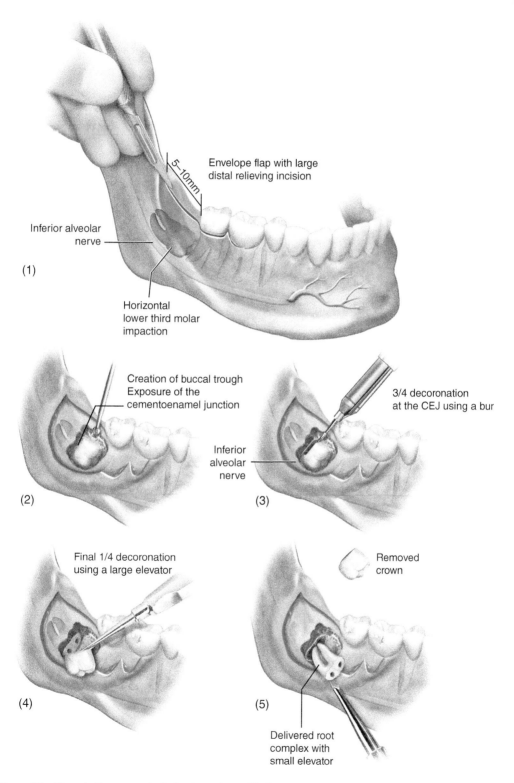

Envelope flap with large
distal relieving incision

5–10mm

Inferior alveolar
nerve

(1)

Horizontal
lower third molar
impaction

Creation of buccal trough
Exposure of the
cementoenamel junction

3/4 decoronation
at the CEJ using a bur

Inferior
alveolar
nerve

(2)

(3)

Final 1/4 decoronation
using a large elevator

Removed
crown

(4)

(5)

Delivered root
complex with
small elevator

Figure 7.5   Steps in the removal of a horizontal mandibular third molar.

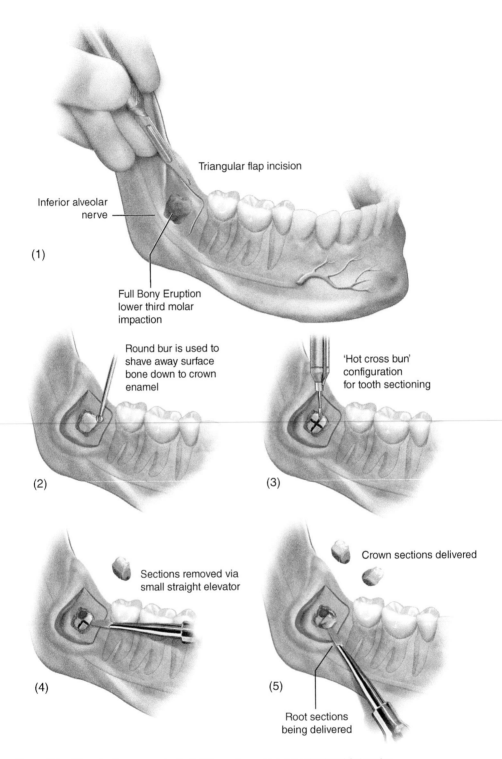

Triangular flap incision

Inferior alveolar
nerve —

(1)

Full Bony Eruption
lower third molar
impaction

Round bur is used to
shave away surface
bone down to crown
enamel

(2)

'Hot cross bun'
configuration
for tooth sectioning

(3)

Sections removed via
small straight elevator

(4)

Crown sections delivered

(5)

Root sections
being delivered

Figure 7.6 Steps in the removal of a full bone impacted mandibular third molar.

7.4.2.4   Full Bony Impaction (Early Root Development)

1) **Soft Tissue Access.** A triangular flap is useful in the context of full bony impacted teeth, as it provides the required access without involving the periodontium of the adjacent teeth. Often, teeth completely submerged in bone teeth do not require extensive bone removal close to the second molar, and as such, soft tissue exposure is not required in this area.

2) **Bone Removal.** In this pattern of third molar impaction, elevation of the flap will expose the body and ramus of the mandible, with no tooth visible. However, the position of the crown of the third molar relative to the second molar can be estimated and measured radiographically. Commence bone removal in a careful and considered manner, in the approximate region of where the third molar crown is predicted to be. A round bur is best suited to this purpose, as it allows bone to be gently shaved away from the surface of the crown, without drilling into the crown itself. Once enamel is seen (or felt through a subtle change in vibration of the handpiece), use a round or fissure bur to expose the occlusal surface of the crown, exposing enough to appreciate the anatomy of the partly formed tooth. The bone window need not be large enough to remove the crown in one piece, as it can instead be sectioned to reduce bone drilling.

3) **Tooth Sectioning.** Divide the crown–root complex into four segments, in a 'hot cross bun' configuration, using a fissure bur (four is usually the minimum number required to produce pieces that can be removed easily from the bony access window). Note that the depth of sectioning need not be as large as in other forms of impacted teeth, as the tooth roots will not have formed as yet, and excessively deep sectioning may result in damage to the surrounding bone and underlying inferior alveolar nerve. Complete tooth sectioning with a Coupland elevator.

4) **Delivery.** Remove the tooth pieces individually, in no particular order, using a small straight elevator. Further sectioning may be required to reduce the size of these pieces for delivery. In some instances, further widening of the bony window can assist in this process. Once each piece of crown has been removed, use a curette to remove any associated follicle and remaining tooth bud.

5) **Cleanup and Closure.** Assess and irrigate the tooth socket to remove any surgical debris. Examine the socket for bleeding, alveolar bone fracture, or soft tissue trauma, and manage as appropriate. Finally, reposition the flap, using a single suture at the corner of the triangular flap, with additional sutures only as necessary (Figure 7.6).

7.4.2.5   Buccolingual/Other Impactions

A wide range of other types of impactions may be clinically indicated for removal. However unique these presentations might be, application of the principles of crown exposure, bone removal, separation of roots to produce individual paths of delivery, and avoidance of vital structures will guide the practitioner. If there is any doubt regarding the likelihood of success of a third molar removal, involvement of a specialist oral and maxillofacial surgeon is indicated.

8

Management of the Medically Compromised Patient

Surgery is the treatment of injuries, conditions, or disorders of the body which require the manipulation, instrumentation, or removal of tissues. However, successful surgery largely depends on the ability of the patient to physiologically cope with surgical stress, as well as the ability of their tissues to undergo postoperative healing. Therefore, thorough consideration must be given to the systemic health of the patient and any underlying medical comorbidities, and how these may influence the outcomes of surgery.

Population ageing has profoundly increased the basic medical knowledge requirements of the contemporary dentoalveolar surgeon. Patient cohorts presenting for dentoalveolar surgery tend to be increasingly frail, have multiple comorbidities, are prescribed several medications, and experience a gradual decrease in organ function and healing ability. These factors place them at an increased risk of developing postoperative complications, and in some cases necessitate avoidance of any surgical procedure. Conversely, the physiologic effects of even minor surgery can cause a profound exacerbation of pre-existing medical illnesses in these groups, leading to sometimes severe and unexpected morbidity.

The presence of serious medical conditions in a patient's medical history warrants a considered discussion with the patient, aiming to answer three key questions:

- What is the effect of the planned surgery on the medical condition?
- What is the effect of the medical condition on the planned surgery?
- How will the associated medications of a medical condition affect the planned surgery?

The list of medical conditions that can influence surgery is extensive. Use of a framework to guide the surgeon in treatment planning will result in safe case selection, a reduced risk of postoperative complications associated with surgery, and ultimately better outcomes for patients.

Common systemic medical conditions implicated in dentoalveolar surgery include:

- Cardiovascular disease.
- Osteoporosis (and medication-related osteonecrosis of the jaws, MRONJ).
- Immunosuppressive conditions (including diabetes mellitus, DM).
- Active or previous head and neck cancer.
- Conditions which require supplemental corticosteroids.
- Bleeding diatheses or conditions requiring anticoagulation.
- Pregnancy.
- Hypertension.

Principles of Dentoalveolar Extractions, First Edition. Seth Delpachitra, Anton Sklavos and Ricky Kumar.
© 2021 John Wiley & Sons Ltd. Published 2021 by John Wiley & Sons Ltd.
Companion website: www.wiley.com/go/delpachitradentoalveolarextractions

This chapter outlines the management of clinical situations in which a medical condition or medication may affect treatment planning in dentoalveolar surgery.

8.1   Ischaemic Cardiovascular Disease

Ischaemic cardiovascular disease is one of the most common groups of conditions encountered in a patient's medical history. A hallmark feature of ischaemic cardiovascular disease is **angina**, chronic intermittent chest pain on exertion that is readily relieved with rest or vasodilatory agents. Severe ischaemic heart disease may present acutely with cardiac arrest due to myocardial infarction. The primary aim of the dentoalveolar surgeon in this group is to prevent the development of an acute cardiac event as a result of any planned surgical procedure.

Patients with a long history of cardiovascular disease or cardiovascular risk factors should be thoroughly assessed for the presence of current symptoms suggestive of uncontrolled disease or unstable ischaemic symptoms. Such patients may experience an acute myocardial infarction triggered by the stress response experience during a dentoalveolar procedure, leading to significant morbidity and, in some cases, death. Elective dental extractions should be avoided in this population group, pending formal assessment and clearance by their treating medical specialist.

Patients with a recent acute ischaemic episode, such as cardiac arrest, myocardial infarction, or a new-onset arrhythmia associated with coronary heart disease, should have any elective dental surgery postponed for at least six months following the event. This includes patients who have had medical or surgical interventions, such as coronary artery bypass grafts or coronary stent angioplasty.

8.2   Patients with a History of Infective Endocarditis

Bacterial colonisation of the endocardial tissues (cardiac valves, chordae tendineae, septal defects) may lead to the development of infective endocarditis. This condition can be acute, occurring on previously normal heart valves as a result of virulent bacteria such as *Staphylococcus aureus*, or subacute, associated with previously abnormal endocardial tissues. Infective endocarditis may result in a number of serious complications, including long-term valvulopathy, systemic spreading infections, and thromboembolic disease.

Any dental procedure, including dentoalveolar surgery, will result in a transient bacteraemia. In the case of prior known valvular abnormality, there is therefore an associated risk of developing infective endocarditis. Antibiotic prophylaxis prior to dentoalveolar extractions may reduce the risk of acute infective endocarditis in high-risk populations. These include patients with:

- A history of infective endocarditis.
- A history of rheumatic heart disease in high-risk groups.
- Previous prosthetic valve repair.
- Cardiac transplant with subsequent valvular disease.
- Congenital heart abnormalities, where:
    - a defect has been fully repaired with prosthetic material in the last six months;
    - a defect has been partially repaired in the past, with exposed prosthetic material; or
    - a defect has been unrepaired, with significant shunting between the left and right atria.

If in any doubt about whether a patient requires antibiotic prophylaxis, specialist clinical advice must be sought from the patient's treating cardiologist.

Guidelines for antibiotic prophylaxis vary internationally, and use of local guidelines and available antibiotics is recommended. Typically, a high 'stat' dose of antibiotic is given prior to the procedure, with enough lead time to allow for maximal systemic absorption before commencement of surgery. Empiric antibiotic choice should be guided by the types of organisms most likely to be involved in bacteraemia from the oral cavity; usually, these belong to the *Streptococcus* spp. group.

8.3 Hypertension

Hypertension is a common condition in the general population. A large number of people require medical management of hypertension, and patients may be on one or more antihypertensive medications, which can affect both dental treatment and the common analgesic choices prescribed after dentoalveolar surgery.

Dental treatment has the unsurprising effect of causing a transient increase in blood pressure. Whilst this is largely innocuous in a healthy individual, acute stress in a hypertensive patient may result in hypertensive crisis: a sudden and severe rise in blood pressure that can result in dizziness, headaches, and nausea, and that rarely can contribute to the development of arrhythmias or haemorrhagic stroke. It is useful to know the patient's most recent blood pressure readings, and to stage procedures to reduce patient stress.

Hypertensive patients are usually on a combination of drugs from a number of classes, including angiotensin-converting enzyme (ACE) inhibitors, angiotensin receptor blockers (ARBs), beta-adrenergic blockers, calcium channel blockers, and diuretic agents. These medications are known to interact with one another and have the propensity to reduce renal function when used in combination with nonsteroidal anti-inflammatory drugs (NSAIDs). The **triple whammy effect** refers to acute ishaemic renal injury caused by the concurrent use of ACE inhibitors or ARBs, diuretics, and NSAIDs. Each of these medications influences renal perfusion through unique mechanisms: ACE inhibitors and ARBs reduce glomerular perfusion pressure through inhibition of vasoconstriction of the efferent arterioles, whilst NSAIDs reduce glomerular perfusion pressure through vasodilatation of the afferent arterioles. When these effects are combined with the volume-depleting effect of diuretics, there is a profound reduction in blood flow through the kidney, resulting in ischaemia and tissue necrosis. The prescription of NSAIDs must be strictly avoided in patients who are using antihypertensive medications.

Hypertensive medications also have the undesirable effect of causing orthostatic hypotension, a posture-related fall in blood pressure. These patients are at an increased risk of syncopal episodes whilst transitioning from a sitting to a standing position. Care should be taken to allow patients time to sit up gently, and assistance should be provided until they are comfortably and safely able to mobilise.

8.4 Medication-Related Osteonecrosis of the Jaws

MRONJ is historically associated with past or current use of antiresorptive medications (Table 8.1). Whilst its presentation is overwhelmingly associated with this group of drugs, other medications have been found to be implicated in its pathophysiology, including antiangiogenic medications and disease-modifying antirheumatic agents.

The clinical presentation of MRONJ can range from unexplained symptoms and radiographic findings to extensive areas of exposed intraoral bone (Figure 8.1) resulting in pathologic fracture,

Table 8.1   Medications associated with the development of MRONJ.

Bisphosphonates	Risendronate
	Alendronate
	Tiludronate
RANKL inhibitors	Denosumab
Antiangiogenics	Bevacizumab
	Sunitinib
Disease-modifying antirheumatic agents (DMARDs)	Methotrexate

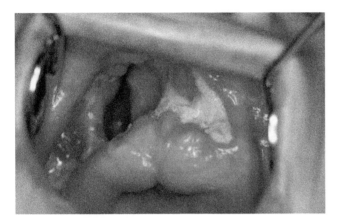

Figure 8.1   Clinical photo of severe and extensive exposed bone from MRONJ, mimicking malignancy. *Source:* Springer Nature.

extraoral draining sinuses, or large oroantral communications (Table 8.2). The diagnosis can be made in patients who have symptoms or signs of MRONJ for a duration of at least eight weeks and a history of past or current antiangiogenic or antiresorptive medication use, in the absence of prior head and neck radiation. The most common initiating factor leading to the development of MRONJ is dentoalveolar surgery, but the condition may also develop as a result of trauma from dental prostheses or odontogenic infection, or occasionally without a known precipitating factor. MRONJ is three times more common in the mandible than the maxilla, likely due to differences in bone vascularity and quality.

The pathophysiology of MRONJ is unclear; it is theorised that the antiosteoclast activity of these agents impairs normal bone turnover, resulting in progressive, nonhealing areas of bone in the oral cavity. It is unknown why the maxilla and mandible are the only bony structures in the body affected by it, but it is conceivable that the complex relationships and functional interactions between bone, tooth, soft tissue, and the oral microbiome play a major role.

The overall population risk of MRONJ in patients exposed to oral bisphosphonate after tooth extraction or other dentoalveolar procedures is approximately 0.5%. The individual risk to each patient is more difficult to predict, as a number of specific factors may influence the incidence of this condition. First, a dose-dependent relationship appears to affect the development of MRONJ; patients who use antiresorptive medications for osteoporosis are generally prescribed a relatively low dose, and thus have a correspondingly low risk of developing MRONJ. Second, the duration of

Table 8.2 American Association of Oral and Maxillofacial Surgery – Clinical Stages of MRONJ.

MRONJ[a] staging	Treatment strategies[b]
At-risk category No apparent necrotic bone in patients who have been treated with either oral or IV bisphosphonates	• No treatment indicated • Patient education
Stage 0 No clinical evidence of necrotic bone, but nonspecific clinical findings, radiographic changes and symptoms	• Systemic management, including the use of pain medication and antibiotics
Stage 1 Exposed and necrotic bone, or fistulae that probe to bone, in patients who are asymptomatic and have no evidence of infection	• Antibacterial mouth rinse • Clinical follow-up on a quarterly basis • Patient education and review of indications for continued bisphosphonate therapy
Stage 2 Exposed and necrotic bone, or fistulae that probe to bone, associated with infection as evidenced by pain and erythema in the region of the exposed bone with or without purulent drainage	• Symptomatic treatment with oral antibiotics • Oral antibacterial mouth rinse • Pain control • Debridement to relieve soft tissue irritation and infection control
Stage 3 Exposed and necrotic bone or a fistula that probes to bone in patients with pain, infection, and one or more of the following: exposed and necrotic bone extending beyond the region of alveolar bone (i.e. inferior border and ramus in the mandible, maxillary sinus, and zygoma in the maxilla) resulting in pathologic fracture, extraoral fistula, oral antral/oral nasal communication, or osteolysis extending to the inferior border of the mandible of sinus floor	• Antibacterial mouth rinse • Antibiotic therapy and pain control • Surgical debridement/resection for longer-term palliation of infection and pain

[a] Exposed or probable bone in the maxillofacial region without resolution for greater than eight weeks in patients treated with an antiresorptive or antiangiogenic agent who have not received radiation therapy to the jaws.
[b] Regardless of the disease stage, mobile segments of bony sequestrum should be removed without exposing uninvolved bone. The extraction of symptomatic teeth within exposed, necrotic bone should be considered since it is unlikely that the extraction will exacerbate the established necrotic process.

therapy appears to be associated with an increased risk, with patients on a bisphosphonate medication for more than three years at a higher risk of developing MRONJ. Third, the type of antiresorptive medication may also influence individual risk. For example, denosumab is only biologically active for approximately four months, after which the risk of MRONJ returns to that of the general population. Bisphosphonates, on the other hand, may maintain biological activity in bone for many years, and patients carry a long-term increased risk of MRONJ even after cessation of medication use. For patients receiving antiresorptive agents for metastatic cancer, multiple myeloma, or hypercalcaemia associated with malignancy, the dose of the drug is significantly higher. These population groups are considered to be high-risk, with a documented risk of MRONJ of up to 15% following dental extraction.

There are several additional contributing factors that can increase the risk of developing MRONJ in patients using antiresorptive or antiangiogenic agents, which tend to be separately associated with poor wound healing. These include DM, tobacco smoking, corticosteroids, poor oral hygiene, and chemotherapeutic agents.

Strategies for the prevention of MRONJ following dental extraction include:

- Risk assessment.
- C-terminal telopeptide (CTX) testing.
- Drug holidays.
- Oral hygiene optimisation.
- An atraumatic extraction technique.

Treatment planning of dentoalveolar extractions in patients at risk of MRONJ requires a case-by-case **risk assessment** and a multidisciplinary approach to the patient's oral and dental care. A comprehensive risk assessment includes a detailed medical history regarding the dose, duration, and type of antiresorptive/antiangiogenic agent, indication for use, other medical conditions, and an assessment of the likely difficulty of extraction and the need for surgical techniques. The indication for tooth extraction must be clear, with all other conservative options considered and expired. Once this information has been gathered and summarised, an informed consent process should occur, outlining whether the patient is in a high-risk category of developing MRONJ and the potential outcomes associated with this condition.

CTX levels are a surrogate marker of bone turnover; a low CTX score implies reduced systemic bone turnover, which may be associated with an increased risk of MRONJ. The validity of the CTX in determining the risk of MRONJ is controversial, and for patients who are symptomatic and require emergency extractions, a CTX test may not be feasible, due to the lead time required for test results to be obtained. Recommendations regarding the interpretation of CTX blood tests prior to elective dentoalveolar surgery are outlined in Table 8.3.

Temporary cessation of an antiresorptive agent, or a **drug holiday**, can be used to minimise the effects of these medications on bone turnover and reduce the risk of MRONJ. The duration of drug holiday required depends on the length of time after administration for which the antiresorptive agent is biologically active. For RANKL inhibitors, this is approximately four months; for bisphosphonate medications, the antiosteoclastic effect can last far longer, depending on the type of bisphosphonate used. The benefits of a drug holiday must be weighed against any risk associated with cessation of the antiresorptive agent, particularly where the indication for use is due to severe osteoporosis or malignancies. Cessation of antiresorptives without consultation with the patient's primary care physician or specialist can result in the development of serious pathologic fracture or worsening of malignant disease. Any decisions regarding drug holidays must be made in a multidisciplinary setting, based on a detailed risk–benefit assessment.

Optimisation of oral hygiene creates a local environment that promotes healing and may reduce the risk of MRONJ. Preoperative periodontal debridement and strict personal oral hygiene should be recommended to the patient in the weeks leading up to dental extraction. Oral hygiene instruction should be continued postoperatively, with the inclusion of a short course of antiseptic mouthwash such as 0.2% aqueous chlorhexidine to reduce oral bacterial load.

Table 8.3 Relative risk of MRONJ based on a C-terminal telopeptide (CTX) blood test, and treatment recommendations.

CTX level	Risk level	Recommendation
<70 µg/l	High	Drug holiday
70–150 µg/l	Moderate	Drug holiday
>150 µg/l	Low	Proceed with extraction

Where possible, the amount of trauma inflicted on the oral tissues during a dental extraction should be minimised – this is commonly referred to as **atraumatic extraction**. Extractions that do not involve the manipulation of soft tissues, avoids bone removal in favour of tooth sectioning, and minimises extraction forces transmitted to the alveolar bone may reduce the risk of development of MRONJ. Obviously, not all teeth can be removed without the use of such techniques; when surgical extraction is indicated, the surgeon must have a level of proficiency and experience sufficient to ensure that the tooth is removed with a reasonable degree of efficiency, and that the soft tissues are managed in a manner conducive to healing. This includes using smaller mucoperiosteal flaps when feasible, minimising tears or trauma to the soft tissues, using a thorough wound toilet with copious sterile saline irrigation, and making an excellent approximation of the soft tissues. For the inexperienced surgeon, difficult cases may be best managed by referral to a specialist or more experienced surgeon.

MRONJ can develop at any stage during the phase of postoperative healing. Following dentoalveolar surgery, at-risk patients require increased postoperative surveillance in the form of regular **follow-up** to assess for mucosal closure. A routine appointment two weeks postoperatively, followed by additional follow-up reviews at six and twelve weeks, will provide sufficient time to review healing and monitor for disease emergence.

Established MRONJ following tooth extraction requires prompt referral to a specialist oral and maxillofacial surgeon for appropriate ongoing medical and surgical management and is outside the scope of this textbook.

8.5   Diabetes Mellitus

'DM' refers to a group of conditions characterised by poor blood glucose control. It may result from an absolute deficiency of insulin due to autoimmune pancreatic disease (type I diabetes) or a relative deficiency of insulin due to tissue insensitivity to the insulin hormone (type II diabetes).

Poorly controlled DM results in poor wound healing and increased risk of infection. As part of the preoperative workup prior to dentoalveolar surgery, the surgeon should acquire as much detail as possible about the individual circumstances regarding the patient's management of their condition. It is recommended that the patient's blood glucose level be tested just prior to the commencement of dentoalveolar surgery – the presence of hypo- or hyperglycaemia may warrant postponement of the surgery until it is appropriately managed. For information regarding the longer-term stability of a patient's blood sugar, a glycosylated haemoglobin (HbA1c) test can be requested from their general physician, although this is less relevant than the blood glucose level in determining whether to proceed with surgery.

Typically, patients with type I DM are managed with supplemental insulin, provided through periodic injections or with an insulin pump. These patients are most commonly susceptible to hypoglycaemic episodes, as dietary fasting without a commensurate reduction in insulin administration may result in excessively low blood sugars. Hypoglycaemia can become a medical emergency, and patients should be specifically informed not to fast prior to dentoalveolar procedures performed under local anaesthetic.

Patients with type II DM may be managed with dietary modification alone, dietary modification with oral hypoglycaemic agents, or the use of supplemental insulin. This group is more likely to develop hyperglycaemia; even in type II diabetics on insulin, hypoglycaemia is rare. Hyperglycaemia is usually asymptomatic, but when severe it may present with nausea, fatigue, diaphoresis, and weakness. In extreme cases, it can be associated with diabetic ketoacidosis, a medical emergency of profound metabolic dysfunction, requiring hospital admission for acute management. If patients present with symptoms suggestive of hyperglycaemia, it is not advisable to proceed with surgery – referral to an appropriate medical service for assessment is recommended.

For patients undergoing extractions under general anaesthetic, specialist medical advice must be sought as to the management of the patient's insulin regime and oral hypoglycaemic agents, as this can be incredibly complex, and varies depending on the timing of the surgery, the type of diabetes, the specific insulin regime, and other systemic factors which may affect blood sugar control. For patients undergoing dental extractions under local anaesthetic, a morning appointment should be offered, and the patient should be counselled on eating normal meals before the procedure. Additionally, oral glucose solutions should be readily available in the clinic, if required – it may be useful to provide these in anticipation of a hypoglycaemic event.

Whilst the risk of postoperative infection is higher in patients with DM, routine antibiotic prophylaxis is not recommended. However, close follow-up is advised, so that any developing or established infections may be treated promptly and aggressively. Routine oral hygiene advice and recommendations for strict blood sugar control may help to reduce the risk of infection.

8.6   Increased Bleeding Risk

Bleeding is an expected but occasionally difficult-to-control complication of any surgical intervention. Even in physiologically normal patients, obtaining haemostasis can be a significant intraoperative challenge; the presence of blood in a surgical site rapidly diminishes both access and vision, making control of a bleeding surgical site or vessel even more difficult.

For patients with an increased tendency to bleed, this is much more of a challenge, and simple methods of haemostasis may not be adequate. Recognition of increased bleeding risk in the preoperative workup is essential in order to reduce unexpected intraoperative complications, achieved through patient optimisation by their primary physician prior to the procedure, preparation of haemostatic adjuncts for use during surgery, and adequate postoperative care and instruction to manage any postoperative haemorrhage.

In general, if there is any suspicion of major or uncontrollable haemorrhage during a dentoalveolar procedure, the patient must be promptly transferred to a tertiary or specialist setting for management. Outpatient and community dental clinics are often not equipped with the staff or training to manage a critical bleed, and this risk is not justified if the surgeon is not in a setting where such complications may be managed.

For patients with increased bleeding risk, it may be wise to restrict the number of teeth to be extracted in a single procedure to three or fewer; a smaller procedure carries a proportionately lower risk. If the patient is having extractions under general anaesthetic, staging of the procedure is not indicated, as this will subject the patient to the risk of multiple general anaesthetics.

Increased bleeding risk may result either from the presence of bleeding diatheses or from the use of medications that affect the physiologic haemostatic process.

8.6.1   Bleeding Diatheses

Several conditions exist which can affect the normal process of haemostasis. These may be congenital, where there is an identifiable genetic cause, or acquired, which have developed as a result of another condition (Table 8.4). Many such conditions are uncommon in the general population, and the diagnosis often remains unknown to the patient. Surgery causing a serious and

Table 8.4 Acquired and congenital conditions which affect normal haemostasis and increase bleeding risk during surgery.

Acquired	Congenital
Vitamin K deficiency	Von Willebrand disease
Liver failure	Haemophilia A, B
Thrombocytopaenia	Idiopathic thrombocytopaenic purpura
	Factor V deficiency
	Factor X deficiency

uncontrollable bleed may be the first time the patient becomes aware of an underlying bleeding disorder. As such, the surgeon must be vigilant in their medical history, in order to identify any family history of bleeding disorders or of other medical conditions which can affect platelet function or the coagulation cascade.

The presence of any of the conditions listed in Table 8.4 warrants involvement of a specialist haematologist prior to any dentoalveolar surgery. Most patients with known coagulopathy will have a dedicated specialist service through which they receive care, with pre-existing management plans should surgery be required. Where possible, referral to a specialist service with both haematology and oral and maxillofacial surgery allows for coordinated care of the patient and appropriate preoperative optimisation.

8.6.2 Medications

Medications which affect haemostasis fall into two major categories: antiplatelet agents and anticoagulants (Table 8.5). Antiplatelet agents inhibit platelet aggregation through interruption of the thromboxane A2–serotonin–ADP positive-feedback cycle involved in platelet activation and aggregation. Anticoagulant agents influence coagulation via inhibition of one or more clotting factors in the coagulation cascade (see Chapter 1).

A variety of medical conditions exist for which these medications may be prescribed, which may carry additional surgical risks that require further precautions to be taken. For example, anticoagulant medications are commonly prescribed for patients with artificial cardiac valves, and antibiotic prophylaxis may be required in these patients prior to major dentoalveolar surgery.

Table 8.5 Common medications which affect normal haemostasis and increase bleeding risk during surgery.

Antiplatelet agents	GPIIb/IIIa inhibitors	Abciximab
		Tirofiban
	ADP inhibitors	Clopidogrel
		Prasugrel
		Ticagrelor
	COX inhibitors	Aspirin
Anticoagulants	Vitamin K antagonist	Warfarin
	Direct factor IIa antagonist	Dabigatran
	Direct factor Xa antagonist	Apixaban
		Rivaroxaban

8.6.2.1 Management of Antiplatelet Agents Prior to Dentoalveolar Surgery

For minor dentoalveolar surgery, antiplatelet agents appear to have only a mild to moderate effect on intraoperative bleeding. This level of bleeding is readily controlled with local haemostatic agents, such as an absorbable packing and suture, as the only modification to the surgical technique. Antiplatelet agents are commonly used in the prevention of stroke and ischaemic cardiovascular disease; cessation of these agents in this cohort will expose the patient to the risk of new stroke or myocardial infarction. As such, it is not recommended that antiplatelet agents be ceased prior to dentoalveolar extractions, as the associated risk for the underlying medical indication exceeds any benefit of the reduction of intraoperative bleeding.

8.6.2.2 Management of Patients Taking Warfarin Prior to Dentoalveolar Surgery

The international normalised ratio (INR) blood test can be used as a surrogate marker of a patient's coagulation function whilst on warfarin. The dose of warfarin, unlike other drugs, varies significantly between patients; as such, obtaining a predictable physiologic effect on an individual patient is dependent on regular INR levels. Additionally, the effect of warfarin on coagulation is highly susceptible to interactions with other drugs or systemic medical conditions that can affect liver metabolism; in such situations, patients may be at excessive bleeding risk despite a previous history of stable anticoagulation. The INR should be checked within 24 hours prior to any dental extractions, to ensure that the patient has sufficient coagulation function for haemostasis after surgery. Generally, it is safe to proceed with dental extraction if the INR is less than 4.0. However, it is still recommended that local haemostatic measures are employed as per the protocol for patients taking anticoagulant medications, including wound packing and suturing, direct pressure with gauze soaked in tranexamic acid solution for at least 30 minutes post-extraction, and use of tranexamic acid mouthwash thrice daily for three to five days following the procedure.

8.6.2.3 Management of Patients Taking Direct Anticoagulant Agents Prior to Dentoalveolar Surgery

Direct factor IIa and Xa antagonists do not require blood monitoring, as their anticoagulant effect is predictable across individuals taking the same dose of medication and approximates that of therapeutic warfarinisation. Whilst there is no blood test that can be reliably used to assess a patient's coagulation function, the current consensus is to manage patients taking direct anticoagulants using the same protocol as for management of patients using warfarin. That is, for minor dentoalveolar surgery, these anticoagulant medications should not be ceased, and local measures should be employed to manage intraoperative or postoperative bleeding. If major dentoalveolar surgery is planned, management of direct anticoagulant medications prior to surgery should occur after consultation with the patient's specialist medical practitioner, or via referral to an oral and maxillofacial surgeon.

8.7 Adrenal Suppression

Glucocorticoids are endogenous hormones produced by the adrenal glands that serve a number of complex physiologic roles in the body. Predominantly, they are known for their powerful anti-inflammatory effects, but they are also involved in sugar, protein, and lipid metabolism, maintenance of blood electrolyte levels, and modulation of tissue growth.

Supplemental glucocorticoids, or corticosteroids, may be prescribed for a number of medical conditions, as listed in Table 8.6.

Table 8.6 Conditions for which corticosteroids are commonly prescribed.

Gastrointestinal	Crohn's disease
	Coeliac disease
	Ulcerative colitis
Respiratory	Asthma
	Chronic obstructive airway disease
Musculoskeletal	Acute muscle or joint injury
	Inflammatory arthritides
Integumentary	Lichen planus
	Vesiculobullous diseases
Vasculitis	Wegener's granulomatosis
	Systemic lupus erythematosus
	Giant cell arteritis
Adrenal	Adrenal insufficiency

Table 8.7 Dose equivalence table for various steroid compositions compared with cortisol.

1 mg cortisol	1 mg hydrocortisone
	0.25 mg prednisolone
	0.04 mg dexamethasone

Part of the physiological response to stress is the production and release of glucocorticoids. Because glucocorticoids are not stored, but rather produced when needed, adrenal suppression by primary insufficiency or by exogenous glucocorticoids will result in the inability of the adrenal glands to produce sufficient steroids to meet physiologic and homeostatic requirements during stress. In such an event, a patient is at risk of developing **adrenal crisis**. Adrenal crisis may present over the following several hours and is characterised by profuse diaphoresis, hypotension, critical electrolyte abnormalities, cyanosis, vomiting, and weakness. If not diagnosed and managed early, it can progress to hypothermia, severe hypotension, hypoglycaemia, confusion, circulatory collapse, and death.

Whilst adrenal crisis is uncommon after dentoalveolar surgery, awareness of this condition and quantification of the risk is necessary in every patient taking regular steroid therapy. For example, not all patients who are taking corticosteroids will have clinically obvious secondary adrenal insufficiency; a longer duration and higher dose are more likely to cause adrenal suppression. Patients using a dose of at least 7.5 mg prednisolone per day (or an equivalent dose of another steroid; see Table 8.7) for at least two weeks appear to be at risk of developing adrenal insufficiency after surgery.

Similarly, greater surgical stress has a higher propensity to result in adrenal crisis. The surgeon should consider this in light of the difficulty of the procedure, age of the patient, any existing infection, and anticipated postoperative pain.

Patients who are at risk of adrenal insufficiency following surgery should be considered for a transient increase in steroid dose in the perioperative period. This should be performed in consultant with their general physician or treating specialist.

8.8 The Irradiated Patient

Radiation therapy in conjunction with surgery is an established treatment modality for head and neck cancer patients. The effects of radiation devastate normal oral physiology, resulting in mucositis in the short term and hyposalivation, caries, periodontal disease, and scarring in the long term.

A critical side effect of radiation to the head and neck is the risk of osteoradionecrosis (ORN) of the jaws. Osteoradionecrosis presents as an area of exposed, devitalised bone that has previously been irradiated which fails to heal over a period of greater than three months in the absence of recurrent neoplastic disease. Irradiated bone is said to become hypoxic, hypocellular, and hypovascular, with a resulting diminished ability to withstand trauma and infection. These conditions are what is thought to precipitate the development of osteoradionecrosis. Furthermore, the risk of osteoradionecrosis is lifelong, and there is no amount of time elapsed after which it is considered 'safe' to remove teeth in the radiation field.

Osteoradionecrosis may occur spontaneously, but there is often an antecedent dentoalveolar injury such as an extraction which precipitates its development. Osteonecrosis has a wide array of severity, from a small asymptomatic area of exposed bone, to extensive exposure associated with pathologic fracture, extraoral fistulae, or lytic lesions involving the nasal and paranasal sinuses. Advanced osteoradionecrosis may require major and lengthy surgical management, including resection and free flap reconstruction, and can pose significant challenges to the patient and their treating medical and surgical teams.

Osteoradionecrosis is predominantly a disease of the mandible, and usually presents in the mandibular body (Figure 8.2). It is most commonly seen in cases where the mandible or maxilla receive a cumulative dose of more than 60 Gray of radiation. A number of other factors contribute to osteoradionecrosis risk, including tumour site and size, malnutrition, poor oral hygiene, and immunosuppression. Surgical extraction of posterior mandible teeth with roots below the mylohyoid line has the highest risk of developing osteoradionecrosis in at-risk groups.

The risk for developing osteoradionecrosis in the past was considerably high, estimated at up to 35%. However, with intensity-modulated radiation therapy and growing awareness about the dental considerations, more recent estimates are lower, with some around 5%.

Patients who have been diagnosed with head and neck cancer are managed by multidisciplinary teams in the hospital setting. Major hospitals may manage all aspects of the patient's treatment, including dentoalveolar extractions, but in rural settings these may be outsourced to public or private dental clinics.

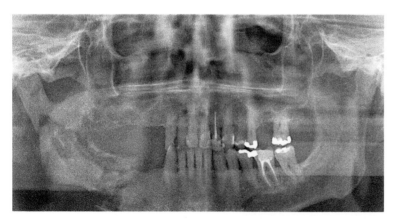

Figure 8.2 Panoramic radiograph of a patient with end-stage osteoradionecrosis causing mandible fracture.

8.8.1 Management of the Patient with a History of Head and Neck Radiotherapy

Hyperbaric oxygen (HBO) therapy has been considered for patients requiring dental extractions and for those with established osteoradionecrosis. The role of HBO is controversial, as there are conflicting results from the various studies conducted on it to date. Therefore, patients who are likely candidates for HBO should be referred to a specialist oral and maxillofacial surgery unit.

Antibiotic prophylaxis may be useful in reducing the risk of development of osteoradionecrosis following dental extractions, but the risk reduction might be as small as 1%. Generally, antibiotic prophylaxis used in osteoradionecrosis is prescribed similarly to that used in infective endocarditis prophylaxis: a single, high-dose antibiotic providing an appropriate spectrum for oral bacteria is prescribed preoperatively. Local guidelines should be employed where a decision to use antibiotic prophylaxis is made.

8.9 Hepatic or Renal Impairment

The liver and kidneys have synergistic functions in the human body, involved in fluid and electrolyte balance, secretion of wastes, hormone production, and overall metabolism. Hepatic or renal impairment can be found in isolation, but in many patients there will be a combination of liver and kidney dysfunctions due to the intimate physiologic relationship between these two organs. There is a litany of medical aetiologies which culminate in the development of hepatorenal impairment, leading to a wide range of clinical presentations of patients in this disease category.

The sequelae of hepatic or renal impairment on patient physiology can be complex and may influence both the decision to proceed with dentoalveolar surgery and the expected postoperative outcomes. Using the framework described at the start of this chapter, outlining the effects of the disease on planned dentoalveolar surgery, outlining the effect of planned surgery on the disease, and recognising the effects of prescribed medication on the surgery is beneficial in such complex conditions (see Table 8.8).

Table 8.8   Considerations in patients with hepatorenal disease undergoing surgery.

Hepatic	Renal
Effect of disease on surgery	
Patient's liver failure may be related to hepatitis B and C, which are communicable diseases	Anaemia of chronic disease may result in a low preoperative haemoglobin level, necessitating specialist management
Postoperative medications require hepatic-adjusted dosing	Postoperative medications require renally adjusted dosing
Antibiotic prophylaxis may be indicated	Antibiotic prophylaxis may be indicated
Patients with advanced liver disease may have an associated coagulopathy, increasing bleeding risk	Hypertension is common, and is usually more severe in patients with a history of renal impairment
Effect of surgery on disease	
Postoperative paracetamol and opiates should be avoided, as these may result in acute liver failure	Postoperative NSAIDs should be avoided, as these may result in acute renal failure
Effect of medications on surgery	
Patients with end-stage hepatic failure may be using a number of medications that can affect surgery	Patients requiring haemodialysis are anticoagulated during and after dialysis, increasing bleeding risk

8.10   Pregnancy and Lactation

When caring for women who are pregnant or lactating, the surgeon should always consider the benefits and risk associated with carrying out a procedure. As a rule, any elective dental treatment, including dentoalveolar surgery, should be postponed until after delivery. Surgical and psychologic stress, postoperative medications, and radiation associated with dental x-rays are best avoided whilst a patient is pregnant.

Dentoalveolar extractions should only be carried out in the pregnant patient if absolutely necessary (e.g. in the case of acute odontogenic abscess). Alternative dental treatments (including endodontic therapy) should be considered, where appropriate. In situations where dental extraction is the only option, referral to a multidisciplinary service with obstetric medicine input is recommended.

9

Postoperative Care and Late Complications

Postoperative care is a critical component of the patient's journey from treatment planning through to completion of extraction therapy. Adequate provision of early postoperative management and sufficient home care instructions, both written and verbal, can significantly reduce the risk of short- and medium-term complications.

9.1 Immediate Postoperative Period

Immediately following completion of a dental extraction, the following procedures must be performed:

- **Adequate Haemostasis of the Surgical Site.** One of the most common presentations following dental extraction is the presence of ongoing bleeding from the surgical site. It is simple to diagnose the cause of post-extraction bleeding in patients with medical comorbidities; in otherwise healthy patients, a more strident approach should be taken. In all patients, regardless of other haemostatic measures utilised during the procedure, simple prevention of surgical-site bleeding can be obtained by immediately placing moist gauze at the site and asking the patient to bite firmly for approximately 10 minutes post-procedure. At the end of the 10-minute period, the gauze should be removed, and the site checked for adequate haemostasis. If bleeding continues, this requires management as outlined in Chapter 6 prior to patient discharge.
- **Temporary Avoidance of Oral Intake or Expectoration.** Following extractions, patients will commonly want to rinse their mouth or expectorate. This can disrupt formation of a stable clot in the fresh extraction socket. It is recommended that patients avoid oral intake, rinsing, or spitting for 30 minutes post-extraction. This needs to be explained to them clearly immediately after removal of haemostatic gauze.
- **Assessment of Patient Wellbeing.** Dental extraction can sometimes be an overwhelming experience for patients. This, combined with their remaining in the supine position for prolonged periods, can lead to postural hypotension or vasovagal syncope in the moments following extraction. A period of rest in the dental chair is recommended to mitigate the risk of fainting. Postural hypotension is much more likely in elderly patients with a history of antihypertensive medication use. Patient wellbeing should be assessed in an informal manner using open-ended questions. Whilst consumption of fluids is a relative contraindication in the first half hour following an extraction, it may be necessary to provide cool water or a glucose drink if the patient feels faint.

Principles of Dentoalveolar Extractions, First Edition. Seth Delpachitra, Anton Sklavos and Ricky Kumar.
© 2021 John Wiley & Sons Ltd. Published 2021 by John Wiley & Sons Ltd.
Companion website: www.wiley.com/go/delpachitradentoalveolarextractions

9.2   Postoperative Instructions

Postoperative instructions should be provided in verbal and written format, and should generally cover the following information:

- **Summary of Procedure Performed.** This should include a list of which teeth were removed and information on whether any changes to the plan of dental extractions were made during the procedure.
- **Open Disclosure Regarding Intraoperative Complications.** Any complications, including damage to other teeth, restorations, or vital structures, should be relayed to the patient. If further surgery or referral is required (e.g. in the case of retained roots or oroantral communication), the patient should be informed of the likely need for repeat surgery with referral to an oral and maxillofacial surgeon.
- **Expected Postoperative Course.** Depending on the number and type of teeth extracted, the normal postoperative course can vary significantly between patients. The patient must be made aware of the expected nature and intensity of any pain, swelling, bruising, or minor bleeding that might occur. Information on home management of these symptoms should also be provided, regarding use of analgesia, ice packs, and jaw rest.
- **Red Flags for Common and Rare Complications.** The patient must be educated on the early warning signs that suggest impending postoperative infection, haematoma, or long-term nerve injury. Early reassessment and appropriate transfer is the key to reducing postoperative morbidity from complications.
- **Planned Reviews and Monitoring.** The patient should be informed of all postoperative follow-up appointments. Generally, in low-risk patients with no medical comorbidities, a one-week planned review is sufficient. In patients with comorbidities or light bleeding risk, a 24-hour review followed by a one-week review ensures early identification of complications.
- **Postoperative Medications and Instructions for Use.** Any postoperative medications prescribed should have clear, written instructions for use.
- **Oral Hygiene and Nutrition Instructions.** Patients may be unsure about how to care for their oral cavity following dental extraction. The pain and nausea associated with surgery may limit oral intake, resulting in dehydration or malnutrition.
- **Self-Care Advice.** Instructions on the avoidance of alcohol and smoking, the need to obtain adequate rest, and the avoidance of exercise can be useful in guiding patients through a smooth recovery period.

9.3   Postoperative Medications

Simple **analgesia** is often sufficient to manage the minor discomfort following dental extraction. Nonsteroidal anti-inflammatory drugs (NSAIDs) tend to work most effectively and are readily available without prescription. Paracetamol (acetaminophen) can be used in conjunction with NSAIDs if additional analgesia is required.

In lieu of saline mouthwashes, an **antiseptic mouthwash** such as aqueous chlorhexidine gluconate 0.2% solution has been shown to reduce the incidence of alveolar osteitis and should be considered in high-risk patients with poor oral hygiene or a history of smoking. Use of chlorhexidine mouthwash should be limited to a maximum duration of two weeks, as it can cause significant tooth discoloration.

There is no evidence for routine prescribing of postoperative **antibiotics** for simple dental extraction. Antibiotics should only be prescribed postoperatively if extraction is being performed as part of the management of an acute odontogenic abscess with facial swelling, or where there is prior evidence of periodontal soft tissue infection with suppuration. Teeth with irreversible pulpitis alone are unlikely to result in acute odontogenic infection following extraction.

9.4   24-Hour On-Call Service and Tertiary Hospital Referral

It is essential that dental practices which offer a dentoalveolar surgery or extraction service provide a 24-hour on-call service or alternative plan in case complications occur out of hours. Rarely, complications of dental extraction may be life-threatening; this can occur at any time following extraction of teeth.

Upon assessment and identification of complications, patients may require transfer to a local oral and maxillofacial surgery department. Every dentoalveolar outpatient clinic should have planned referral pathways to the local hospital to facilitate this transfer as required. Verbal and written communication with a clinician in the receiving department is an important component of safe and appropriate patient handover.

9.5   Management of Late Complications

Whilst the list of intraoperative complications following dental extraction is extensive, there are fewer late complications that can occur. These are equally important, however, as they are the main reason that patients seek unplanned emergency treatment, which may occur out of hours. Patients may present in an unpredictable or delayed manner, and the surgeon must be well prepared to manage complications that require urgent treatment or hospital transfer.

9.5.1   Alveolar Osteitis

Alveolar osteitis, colloquially referred to as 'dry socket', occurs when the fibrin clot in the extraction socket is not maintained, resulting in an empty tooth socket exposed to the oral environment. The typical presentation will be severe pain developing 48 hours after a dental extraction procedure, associated with halitosis and malaise. Alveolar osteitis is not an infection per se, and so findings of fluctuance, vestibular swelling, discharge, or facial abscess are not associated with an isolated dry socket.

This condition is more common in females, usually occurs with extraction of mandibular molar teeth, and has an association with use of the oral contraceptive pill, poor oral hygiene, and smoking.

All patients should be advised of the risk of a dry socket developing after any dental extraction. Overall, the risk is approximately 5%, but patients should be advised that this may be higher when they have one or multiple risk factors present.

Management of alveolar osteitis includes pharmacological treatment with analgesia and chlorhexidine mouthwash and placement of an antiseptic or analgesic dressing such as Alvogyl. Alvogyl combines iodoform, eugenol, and butamben in a fibrous, nonabsorbable paste which has anaesthetic and antiseptic properties and typically provides immediate relief. Patients who have been treated with any dressing with a fibrous or nonresorbable component should be reviewed within 48 hours for its removal; left *in situ*, such a dressing may become a nidus of infection, requiring evacuation.

Surgical debridement and washout of the socket under local anaesthesia is another appropriate management strategy for alveolar osteitis, as this allows for removal of any debris and promotes formation of a new clot. However, this may cause additional discomfort to an already disconcerted patient, who will often opt against any further surgical intervention in the short term.

9.5.2 Acute Facial Abscess

Dentoalveolar extractions create an intraoral wound which is susceptible to developing infection. Postoperative infections will present with the cardinal signs of inflammation: swelling, redness, pain, and heat, and associated purulent discharge from the surgical site. Such infections may be small localised collections or a serious life-threatening infection involving deep spaces in the head and neck, leading to airway compromise and trismus.

Patients who have undergone dental extractions should always be provided with a postoperative plan which outlines what to do if a developing infection is suspected. At minimum, this should include urgent review by the treating surgeon.

On review, patients should be assessed for trismus, dysphagia, odynophagia, mouth opening, impending upper airway obstruction, and signs of systemic infection. Their oral intake should be assessed and a clinical examination should be undertaken to determine the extent of the swelling. Important features to note are swelling in the floor of the mouth or that which is firm and crosses the border of the mandible, any parapharyngeal bulging or deviation of the uvula from the midline, and any infection spreading and causing periorbital cellulitis.

Clinical signs and symptoms will dictate the appropriate management for patients who develop a postoperative infection. Infections of the buccal space, with swelling of the cheek and vestibule, generally tend to be minor and to be amenable to intraoral incision and drainage under local anaesthetic. Infections involving the submandibular or sublingual spaces tend to be more severe and much more likely to result in airway compromise – these always require hospital admission and a combination of intra- and extraoral drainage. Radiographic investigation will help determine the possible cause. For example, a patient might develop an infection due to a retained root, bone sequestra, or a foreign body (dressings or other materials).

The presence of facial swelling with suspicion of abscess warrants immediate surgical intervention. Antibiotic therapy alone is not appropriate management for acute facial abscesses. The development of an abscess is a late sign of infection, and therefore surgical incision and drainage of the abscess, with washout of the involved fascial spaces, is the mainstay of management of this condition. Antibiotics are a useful adjunct treatment for managing the associated facial cellulitis, but are ineffective against mature, walled-off collections of pus.

Patients who develop severe infections with signs of airway compromise, fever, or trismus preventing oral intake require prompt referral via ambulance to a hospital-based oral and maxillofacial surgery service, where appropriate medical and surgical management can be initiated. These patients may progress to develop infections that involve deeper neck or thoracic spaces, requiring tracheostomy, multiple washout procedures, and a lengthy stay in an intensive care unit.

An acute facial infection may herald the development of osteomyelitis of the jaw: a catastrophic deep infection of the maxillary or mandibular bone. This is typically a disease of immunocompromised patients but can sometimes occur in healthy individuals. Early signs of osteomyelitis resemble those of acute odontogenic or postoperative infections and can be difficult to differentiate in the earlier stage of the disease process. Acute osteomyelitis can result in the accumulation of purulent discharge under the periosteum, with an associated periosteal reaction visible on radiographic imaging. The associated mucosa and skin are usually erythematous and very tender to palpation, with discharge from multiple intra- and extraoral fistulae. Osteomyelitis may also cause paraesthesia when the infection is present around the inferior alveolar canal. Radiographic features suggestive of osteomyelitis include a moth-eaten appearance with presence of large sequestra. Immediate referral to a hospital infectious diseases unit is recommended.

9.5.3 Postoperative Haemorrhage

Postoperative haemorrhage may present within the first few days after dentoalveolar extraction. Unlike with intraoperative haemorrhage, patients will already have been discharged, under the presumption that all bleeding has been adequately controlled. A slow postoperative haemorrhage can lead to significant blood loss; as patients are not under observation at home, occult bleeding may be missed, and it may be very late in the picture before they seek medical assistance.

There are two forms of postoperative bleeding in healthy patients: delayed primary bleeding and secondary bleeding. Delayed primary bleeding occurs within the first several hours post-dental extraction, and is caused by the waning of the vasoconstrictive effect of local anaesthetics. Secondary bleeding occurs days after extraction, and is usually related to infection producing an inflammatory and vasodilatatory response in the local tissues.

In the assessment of any patient with postoperative haemorrhage, the primary survey must be undertaken to assess their cardiovascular status and estimated blood loss. Large haemorrhages may cause haemodynamic compromise, which itself requires transfer to a local hospital service for resuscitation. Once the patient has been deemed to be haemodynamically stable, attempts should be made using local methods to control the bleeding (see Chapter 6). Simultaneously, the patient's history should be revisited in order to determine any systemic medical conditions which might have contributed to the onset of the bleed. The patient should also be examined for any signs of developing soft tissue infection; if this is a potential cause of haemorrhage, antibiotic therapy may be indicated.

Once haemostasis has been achieved, the patient requires close follow-up after 24 hours and then after one week, to ensure that bleeding has subsided and any causes have been identified and managed appropriately.

9.5.4 Temporomandibular Joint Disorder

Temporomandibular joint disorders (TMDs) are common in the general population; a considerable proportion of patients presenting for dentoalveolar extractions will have pre-existing TMD. This should be documented in the patient history, and a comprehensive temporomandibular joint assessment should form part of the preoperative workup, including a record of maximal mouth opening, joint crepitus, hypermobility, locking, and pain on movement. It is uncommon to develop TMD *de novo* following dental extraction procedures; usually, there will be some evidence suggesting subclinical temporomandibular joint disease.

Patients with TMD may experience an exacerbation of their condition after extractions. This is largely due to the force applied to the joint and masticatory musculature during mandibular extractions, but it can be also related to prolonged mouth opening during maxillary ones. An efficient and safe operator is much less likely to cause TMD; appropriate and effective use of forces, early determination of the need for surgical extraction, and timely use of patient breaks between longer procedures prevent inadvertent stress on the temporomandibular joint.

Patients who develop symptoms of TMD following extraction will be understandably concerned regarding the onset of such syndromes. A full assessment and diagnosis should be undertaken to rule out other causes of temporomandibular symptoms. If the patient's presentation can be explained by intraoperative trauma or a prolonged and forceful procedure, the prognosis is generally good, and there will likely be a return to baseline after three months postoperatively. Advice on conservative management (including jaw rest, physiotherapy, and anti-inflammatory medications) should be provided, with regular follow-up to assess for clinical improvement. Rarely, patients may require advanced management by an oral medicine specialist or oral and maxillofacial surgeon, and a timely referral may be required.

9.5.5 Epulis Granulomatosa

The normal healing of an extraction socket involves the formation of granulation tissue inside it, which is gradually replaced by bone and gingival soft tissue. This normal healing may be complicated by the development of hyperplastic granulation tissue that exudes out of the socket and into the oral cavity, giving the appearance of an epulis (Figure 9.1). This is usually a foreign-body reaction to debris or bony sequestra in the socket, as a result of inadequate debridement following extraction. Occasionally, haemostatic dressings or treatments used for alveolar osteitis may be implicated in this reaction.

Epulis granulomatosa is clinically indistinguishable from intra-alveolar squamous cell carcinoma or other giant cell lesions of the jaws. As such, the presence of this hyperplastic tissue warrants urgent biopsy for formal histopathologic diagnosis. Simultaneous curettage and debridement of the socket is often adequate to treat epulis granulomatosa and encourage normal healing.

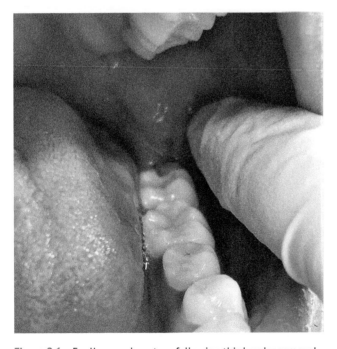

Figure 9.1 Epulis granulomatosa following third molar removal.

9.5.6 Nerve Injury

Extraction of mandibular teeth carries the risk of iatrogenic injury to branches of the mandibular division of the trigeminal nerve: specifically, the inferior alveolar nerve; its terminal branch, the mental nerve; and the lingual nerve. These nerves have close anatomic relations to the mandible and associated dentition, as they provide sensation to these structures. Nerve injury commonly results from direct intraoperative trauma during the dental extraction procedure. It may also result from complications related to local anaesthetic injection, but this is generally less likely.

The incidence of nerve injury is normally considered to be quite low. Amongst such injuries, most will be a temporary paraesthesia which usually resolves after weeks to months. Permanent paraesthesia is less common, with an incidence of less than 1%. A more unfavourable but less likely scenario is dysaesthesia, the development of a painful or unpleasant sensation in the distribution of the nerve. It is important to note that published nerve injury rates are highly variable and not applicable to individual surgeons, as they do not always take into account caseload difficulty, operator experience, and site-specific guidelines for management of high-risk cases.

Nerve injuries may be considered as neuropraxia, axonotmesis, or neurotmesis. This distinction is based on the extent of injury and gives an important indication of the likelihood of recovery.

- **Neuropraxia** refers to situations where the nerve sheath has been traumatised but there is no axonal injury. This is the mildest form of injury, typically from minor compression or traction. The result is a partial or complete conduction block, which will present as a paraesthesia in the distribution of the nerve. The prognosis of neuropraxia is excellent, with total recovery of nerve function within three months post injury.
- **Axonotmesis** occurs when more severe damage has occurred to the nerve sheath, with associated partial axonal disruption. The prognosis is unpredictable, and there may be only partial recovery of nerve function, with potential for long-term dysaesthesia. Recovery of nerve function may take months to years.
- **Neurotmesis** is the most severe form of injury, and occurs when the nerve has been completely transected, with loss of continuity of the axon. This is typically due to direct trauma to the nerve through contact with sharp surgical instruments or due to inadvertent stretching and tearing. There will be minimal to no recovery of nerve function without surgical repair. Furthermore, recovery will be complicated by Wallerian degeneration and the development of a traumatic neuroma at the transected nerve end, leading to chronic neuropathic pain.

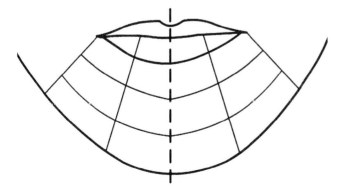

Figure 9.2   Nerve map used for identification and follow-up of injuries to the inferior alveolar nerve.

A routine component of surgical follow-up after extraction of mandibular teeth should be an assessment of lingual and inferior alveolar nerve function. This will often be something that the patient raises without prompting, as it has a notable effect on quality of life. If there is suspicion or clinical indication of nerve injury, objective and repeatable assessment is required in order to assess its severity; this will act as a baseline against which future assessments can be compared in determining improvement or change. One of the simplest methods of assessment is nerve distribution mapping, using predetermined anatomic landmarks to assess on a scale of 1–10 the extent of paraesthesia (Figure 9.2). Any disruption to the sensation of taste should also be documented.

Once baseline measurements have been obtained, the patient should be reviewed after four weeks, repeating the same nerve mapping documentation. Early and marked improvement in nerve scoring is a good indication that the patient will have a complete recovery of nerve function. In the event that there is little or no improvement within three months, or where at baseline the sensation is reported as 0 across the entire distribution of the nerve, the patient may benefit from a specialist opinion from an oral and maxillofacial surgeon, for further assessment and consideration of surgical nerve repair.

Appendix A

Special Cases: Common Indications for Surgical Extraction

A.1 Lone-standing Upper First Molars

The lone-standing upper first molar can be one of the more difficult teeth to extract. This is a common presentation in older adults, where the first molar is the oldest (and often the last posterior tooth) left in the arch. It is typical that the periodontal ligament space is much smaller as a result of a lifetime of functional cycles occurring on the tooth. Additionally, roots may be splayed and a pneumatised sinus lining can extend right to the furcation of the tooth. Simple extraction of upper first molars is ill-advised in these situations, due to the propensity to cause large oroantral communication. A lower threshold should exist for surgical sectioning and root removal.

A crestal mucoperiosteal flap must be raised with mesial and distal relieving incisions, and the buccal surface of the crown exposed. Bone removal should be performed as judiciously as is required to expose the cementoenamel junction, but no further. The crown should be decoronated to expose the pulp chamber and visualise the root anatomy, and the roots sectioned, being careful not to drill deeper than the tooth furcation, given the proximity of the sinus lining. Once sectioned, the palatal, mesiobuccal, and distobuccal roots can be gently delivered using a small, straight elevator. Prior to closure, it is wise to examine for the presence of an oroantral communication and manage as necessary.

A.2 Palatally Impacted Upper Canines

Removal of impacted maxillary canines is an advanced dentoalveolar surgery skill. Upper canines may be indicated for removal in adolescents or young adults as part of a larger orthodontic treatment plan, or in older adults where there is associated pathology (e.g. adjacent root resorption or odontogenic tumours). Palatally impacted upper canines pose a unique challenge due to limitations in access, the need for a large palatal flap, the presence of surrounding anatomic structures (including tooth roots and the nasal and paranasal sinuses), and the density and volume of bone that may require removal in order to access the tooth.

A number of serious complications can occur with removal of palatally impacted upper canines. Excessive bone removal from the palate may lead to the inadvertent creation of an oronasal or oroantral communication, which can become a chronic functional problem necessitating advanced surgical repair. Consideration of the three-dimensional position of the maxillary tooth roots is essential; damage to the periodontal ligaments or apices of adjacent maxillary teeth may lead to

Principles of Dentoalveolar Extractions, First Edition. Seth Delpachitra, Anton Sklavos and Ricky Kumar.
© 2021 John Wiley & Sons Ltd. Published 2021 by John Wiley & Sons Ltd.
Companion website: www.wiley.com/go/delpachitradentoalveolarextractions

ankylosis or loss of vitality. Failure to properly elevate and mobilise the tooth remnants can result in displacement of components into the nasal or paranasal sinuses, requiring a salvage procedure.

Preoperative planning is essential prior to attempting removal of an impacted maxillary canine. Localisation and visualisation of the surrounding structures is best obtained with a cone-beam computed tomography (CBCT) scan. This will guide the surgeon as to the precise location of the tooth, and vector of the root for extraction. Plain-film occlusal radiographs combined with periapical views have been used for localisation, but these are largely superseded in the age of readily available, low-cost, low-dose CBCT.

Profound local anaesthetic of the entire palate is essential for this often challenging procedure - more often than not, surgeons will prefer general anaesthetic given the difficulties in access and anaesthesia. Bilateral greater palatine blocks, with buccal infiltration of the maxillary canine region, provide patient comfort and tolerance.

The procedure should commence by raising a generous crestal flap from the ipsilateral first molar to the contralateral canine region. Sufficient exposure is critical to provide access to the entire pericoronal bone of the canine. The robust keratinised mucosa of the palate is readily elevated in the subperiosteal plane. Care should be taken to avoid injuring the incisive nerve, which lies approximately 5 mm posterior to the midline of the maxillary alveolus.

Bone removal can be commenced in a routine fashion, to expose the entire crown to the cementoenamel junction. In situations where the canine is completely bony impacted and not visible, great care should be taken to only drill bone where the crown is predicted to be closest to the palate.

Once the crown is exposed, its sectioning and removal will provide access to the long single root. This remaining root can be sectioned axially and removed in pieces.

When cleanup and haemostasis is achieved, closure may be performed by repositioning of the palatal flap and suturing using interdental sutures at the papillae.

A.3 Bulbous Roots (Hypercementosis)

Bulbous roots represent a unique dentoalveolar challenge. Hypercementosis is a process by which additional cementum is laid down along the roots of lone-standing teeth, resulting in roots that may be wider at the apical area compared to the coronal area. Bulbous roots defy conventional practicalities of tooth removal, where roots are normally cone-shaped and are delivered along a standard vector of extraction. However, the general principles of extraction still apply: a clear vector of delivery should be planned, and sufficient space should be created to deliver the root in parts or whole. Often, bone removal to the level of the widest part of the tooth is not a viable or wise option, if maintenance of the alveolar process for future implants is a consideration. However, this may still be required if axial sectioning is likely to be difficult.

Following anaesthesia, an appropriate flap should be raised to provide sufficient access to the alveolar process of the tooth to be extracted. Sufficient bone should be removed along the alveolus adjacent to the tooth to expose the root structure past the cementoenamel junction. Decoronation as an early step is essential to visualise the bulbous tooth root at that junction.

Once the tooth root has been isolated, a decision must be made as to whether axial sectioning of the root will be attempted or deeper bone removal is required. This decision should ideally be made preoperatively, based upon the vertical location of the thickest part of the root; however, the large variability in pattern and presentation of hypercementosis may dictate an intraoperative change to the surgical approach. A combination of approaches could be required in order to deliver the whole tooth.

If the unfortunate circumstance occurs where the root fractures low, above the area of hypercementosis, then a large buccal bony window will be required in order to remove the whole tooth. Careful consideration should be taken regarding the long-term health of the alveolus if significant bone removal is required, as this can impact future dental rehabilitation.

A.4 Teeth with Aberrant Root Morphology

Whilst in most cases the root formation of a tooth is predictable, there are several situations in which the number of roots, and the root anatomy, may deviate from what is expected. Examples include:

- **Abnormally Multirooted Teeth.** Most commonly, canine teeth with two roots.
- **Root Dilacerations.** Sudden deviations in the angulation of a root.
- **Taurodontism.** Apical displacement of the tooth furcation.

The presence of aberrant root morphology is not always appreciable clinically, and it warrants close radiographic examination and surgical planning prior to commencement of tooth extraction. Failure to detect aberrant root morphology, particularly in dilacerated teeth, can lead to intraoperative root fracture at the level of the dilaceration, making removal of the fragment extremely difficult. Surgical extraction, involving flap elevation, tooth sectioning, and generous bone removal, is nearly always required; this should be discussed with the patient, and their consent obtained.

Key to the successful and total removal of a tooth with aberrant root morphology is identification of the vectors for extraction of each individual root fragment. Canine teeth with clearly separate multiple roots must be treated similarly to premolar teeth; each root must be treated as having separate exit paths, and the tooth must be sectioned to deliver each separately. Similarly, teeth exhibiting taurodontism generally require a deep sectioning as close to the furcation as possible, and this necessitates a large bone gutter in order to access the apical portion of the root.

Dilaceration poses a particularly difficult dilemma, even in single-rooted teeth, as the acute deviation of the tooth root does not permit a clearly identifiable vector of tooth removal. Whilst removal of the crown is often required in order to visualise the root and remove interferences, sectioning within a dilacerated root is ill-advised, as maintenance of a point of elevation is essential to allow for socket expansion and root mobilisation. Creation of a straight exit path may usually be achieved with controlled but extensive bone removal towards the inner line angle of the root where there is a change of angle. This will allow the root to be gently elevated and delivered around the curvilinear vector that has been created.

A.5 Teeth with Extensive Crown Decay

Subgingival or extensive crown decay may be an immediate preoperative indication for surgical techniques for tooth removal. Efficient application of elevators or extraction forceps requires a stable contact point between the tooth and alveolar bone; the presence of caries significantly increases the risk of crown fracture, instrument slippage, and application of undue and uncontrolled force on adjacent teeth.

In many circumstances, this difficulty in application of force is due to an inability to visualise the periodontal ligament space between the tooth and the bone. Simple elevation of a flap may be all that is required to identify a required application point for a luxator. If, after elevation, the root caries extend too close to the alveolar bone level, bone removal may help expose sound dentine of the roots, as well as create space for application of the elevator. Tooth sectioning should be used judiciously for multirooted teeth, to facilitate safe elevation of each root along its own axis.

A.6 Retained Deciduous Molars

Retained deciduous molar teeth may pose a deceptively challenging scenario for tooth extraction. They usually result from the absence of a permanent successor. As the permanent dentition erupts into the mouth, ankylosis results in submergence of the primary tooth below the occlusal plane. Often, the deciduous tooth is tightly wedged between the convex cementoenamel surfaces of the two adjacent teeth, making application of forceps and conventional dental extraction impossible. Further, the thin and comparatively weak roots of the deciduous teeth are generally ankylosed to the underlying bone, and incomplete removal of roots due to crown fracture may require extensive bone removal. This must be avoided, or at least minimised, in situations where subsequent implant restoration is planned – which is normally the case, as patients presenting for removal of ankylosed deciduous teeth are often doing so in order to facilitate implant placement.

Removal of a retained deciduous molar should begin with elevation of a generous mucoperiosteal flap, in order to visualise the tooth–bone interface and estimate the position of the furcation of the tooth. At this point, no buccal bone removal is recommended. Instead, the crown of the tooth should be sectioned within the alveolus with a fissure bur to the estimated depth of the furcation. A Coupland's No. 2 gouge may be placed in between the mesial and distal halves of the tooth, and the section very gently completed. Care should be taken not to place excessive force through the crown at this stage, as root fractures may commonly occur.

Once the mesial and distal halves of the tooth are mobilising independently, the elevator can be placed into the interproximal areas mesial and distal to the deciduous molar, gently luxating the crown–root complexes towards the section. Finally, each half may be removed from the socket using root forceps.

Appendix B

Extraction of Deciduous Teeth

Paediatric dental patients pose a number of unique challenges compared with the adult population. Fundamentally, however, the principles and techniques employed in the extraction of paediatric teeth are similar to those used in adults. Indications of tooth extraction must be based upon a sound history, examination, and investigation. Any procedure must take into account the patient and their overarching dental treatment plan. The age of the patient and their stage of dental development may influence how deciduous extraction sites are managed as their permanent successors erupt into the space.

B.1 Principles of Paediatric Dental Extraction

B.1.1 History Taking and Examination

The history taken prior to removal of teeth from a paediatric patient must be obtained from both the child and their attending parent or carer. The age of the patient and their stage of psychosocial and cognitive development will have a significant influence on what extraction treatment is required, how much treatment can be provided in a single session, and what behavioural and pharmacologic behaviour management strategies must be employed. In particular, the child's behaviour during the initial assessment will guide the surgeon as to whether extraction can be easily provided under local anaesthetic in the dental chair, or whether additional forms of sedation (e.g. relative analgesia, general anaesthesia) are required. Use of communication and behaviour management techniques should be tailored to the individual patient's developmental stage. Examination of the patient's mouth should be comprehensive, in order to account for any other treatment that is required in addition to dental extraction. Extensive treatment may present an indication for general anaesthetic rather than requiring multiple lengthy visits, which might reduce patient acceptance of dental treatment.

B.1.2 Radiographic Assessment

A deciduous tooth that appears clinically indicated for extraction must be assessed radiographically in the same way as an adult tooth. In children, a periapical radiograph or orthopantomogram is sufficient to examine the root morphology and crown integrity prior to extraction. Paediatric

Principles of Dentoalveolar Extractions, First Edition. Seth Delpachitra, Anton Sklavos and Ricky Kumar.
© 2021 John Wiley & Sons Ltd. Published 2021 by John Wiley & Sons Ltd.
Companion website: www.wiley.com/go/delpachitradentoalveolarextractions

patients under the age of five may not be suitable for orthopantomographic imaging due to the behavioural requirements of this form of radiograph, but it can be useful for examining the overall dentition and the stage of dental development.

B.1.3   Consent

In many jurisdictions worldwide, consent for treatment concerning patients under the age of 18 falls to the patient's parent or legal guardian. The consent process should nonetheless involve obtaining informed consent from all parties, taking care to explain the procedure, indications, risks, benefits, and alternatives to the patient as well as their carer. Patients under the age of 18 may be deemed to be 'Gillick competent'; that is, sufficiently able to understand the treatment being provided and its attendant risks and expected outcomes. The surgeon must be well versed in local laws and regulations regarding medical treatment of minors and the consent process involved.

B.1.4   Local Anaesthetic

In paediatric patients, local anaesthetic serves primarily to manage intraoperative pain during dental extraction, but it also acts as an important behaviour-modification strategy in eliminating any external response or resistance to dental treatment. Local anaesthetic strategies in the paediatric population differ significantly from those used with adults:

- **Dose.** The relative low body mass compared with adults corresponds to a lower total dose of local anaesthetic that may be administered. Whilst the dose per kilogramme of body weight remains the same between child and adult, the absolute volume of any given concentration of anaesthetic will be much lower.
- **Duration of Anaesthetic.** Long-acting local anaesthetics are not recommended in younger paediatric groups. Uncontrolled lip biting after local anaesthetic administration can lead to significant soft tissue trauma and is commonly seen after the use of long-acting agents such as bupivacaine. Therefore, only short-acting agents such as lignocaine should be used in the paediatric patient, in order to avoid this complication.
- **Techniques.** Due to the porous nature of maxillary and mandibular bone in children, buccal and palatal/lingual infiltration may be sufficient to obtain anaesthesia for deciduous dental extractions in patients under the age of six. Use of inferior alveolar nerve blocks may be required for the removal of mandibular teeth in patients older than this.

B.1.5   Use of Sedation

In addition to local anaesthetic, a ladder of anaesthetic interventions is available to improve a child's tolerance of a dental procedure. Conscious sedation, employing nitrous oxide administered via a nasal hood, is commonly available in the dental clinic setting and is a safe method of obtaining patient comfort without loss of consciousness or pharyngeal and laryngeal reflexes. Oral sedation, intravenous sedation, and general anaesthesia may also be utilised, depending on the level of behaviour modification required and the complexity of treatment. Whilst a further discussion on the merits, indications, and techniques of sedation is outside the scope of this manual, provision of these services must be made by appropriately trained personnel, in a setting which is sufficiently prepared to manage any associated complications.

Table B.1   Options for space maintenance after deciduous tooth extraction.

Band/crown-loop
Distal shoe
Lingual holding arch
Palatal/transpalatal arch
Nance appliance
Removable appliance
Bonded space maintainer

B.1.6   Extraction Technique

The extraction technique for deciduous extractions differs from that for adult teeth:

- Generally, less force is required to rupture the periodontal ligament.
- Adjacent teeth are more likely to be inadvertently luxated or avulsed if elevators or forceps are applied incorrectly.
- Paediatric bone is more elastic than adult bone, and expansion of the socket is easier.
- Root anatomy is more predictable (incisors and canines have straight, conical roots; deciduous molars have a mesial and distal root).
- Deciduous tooth roots are thinner and root fracture is more likely.
- Retrieval of fractured roots carries the risk of damage to the crown and follicle of the developing succedaneous tooth.
- Submerged or ankylosed deciduous teeth in adults will almost always require surgical methods for extraction, due to fusion of thin roots to the underlying bone.

B.1.7   Outcomes Following Extraction

Extraction of a deciduous tooth generally occurs before that tooth has reached the appropriate timing for exfoliation. There are a number of potentially negative sequelae that may follow early loss of a deciduous tooth, including arch asymmetry, reduced arch length, ectopic eruption of permanent teeth, and midline discrepancies. In conjunction with specialist paediatric dentists, a clear plan must be put in place for space maintenance following tooth extraction, to facilitate continued normal dental development and avoidance of complications (Table B.1).

- Premature loss of anterior teeth (incisors and canines) can cause loss of space due to a lateral shift of the other anterior teeth, causing a midline discrepancy. This is most pronounced if a primary canine tooth is extracted or lost early. Loss of space does not tend to occur after removal of a primary incisor, so long as the primary canine is fully erupted.
- Premature loss of posterior teeth can cause distal movement of the primary canine and incisors, as well as mesial eruption of the first permanent molar. This space loss is greatest if the first permanent molar has not completed eruption, and tends to be worse in the maxilla than the mandible.

B.2   Techniques of Paediatric Dental Extraction

B.2.1   Deciduous Incisors and Canines

1) **Difficulty Assessment.** Deciduous incisors and canines are straight-rooted teeth. It is extremely rare to require surgical techniques for extraction of teeth in this category. Root

resorption due to eruption of underlying permanent teeth generally reduces the amount of force required to extract a deciduous incisor or canine.

2) **Consent.** General risks of dental extraction apply. Damage to underlying permanent teeth is always a risk of deciduous tooth extraction and must be explicitly included in the consent process. Space maintenance plans should be included in the consent process.

3) **Basic Equipment.** Paediatric upper straight forceps are used for maxillary incisors and canines, and paediatric lower universal forceps for mandibular ones. A straight elevator should be available to expand the periodontal ligament prior to forceps placement.

4) **Final Check.** The tooth number and location must be confirmed on radiograph.

5) **Local Anaesthetic.** Infiltration of the buccal vestibule with localised palatal (for maxillary teeth) or lingual (for mandibular teeth) infiltration will provide sufficient anaesthesia for the soft tissue and periodontal ligament.

6) **Positioning.** The patient should be positioned lying almost flat, with the patient's head and headrest slightly raised.

7) **Elevation.** A straight elevator should be applied to the mesial and distal areas of the periodontal ligament. Using a wheel-and-axle motion, the periodontal ligament should be gently expanded until a small amount of mobility is noted in the tooth. Care must be taken to elevate between tooth and bone only, and not against adjacent teeth. The thumb and finger of the non-dominant hand should be used to support the alveolus of the tooth being extracted, to guide the application of force to the tooth socket only, and to prevent instrument slippage.

8) **Delivery.** The forceps should be applied to the cementoenamel junction. Initially, apical pressure is used to slide the beaks as deep on to the root as possible. Rapid, small clockwise–counterclockwise rotational movements should then be used to continue tearing the periodontal ligament. Finally, the buccal part of the crown should be rotated towards the midline.

9) **Assessment.** The tooth root should be assessed to ensure it has been removed complete. The socket must be examined for bleeding, alveolar bone fracture, or soft tissue trauma, which should be managed as appropriate. Instrumentation of the socket should be avoided, as the underlying permanent tooth may be damaged.

B.2.2 Deciduous Molars

1) **Difficulty Assessment.** Both maxillary and mandibular deciduous molars have a predominantly mesial and distal root configuration. Depending on the stage of dental development, there may be significant resorption of the tooth roots due to eruption of the underlying permanent tooth. This can increase the likelihood of root fracture during extraction. In general, root fracture is common during removal of a deciduous molar tooth.

2) **Consent.** General risks of dental extraction apply. Damage to underlying permanent teeth is always a risk of deciduous tooth extraction and must be explicitly included in the consent process. Space maintenance plans should be included in the consent process.

3) **Basic Equipment.** Paediatric upper molar forceps are used for maxillary molars, and paediatric lower molar forceps for mandibular ones. Adult forceps are not recommended for use in paediatric populations as there is poor adaptation of the forceps beaks to the teeth, increasing the risk of root or crown fracture. A straight elevator should be available to expand the periodontal ligament prior to forceps placement.

4) **Final Check.** The tooth number and location must be confirmed on radiograph.

5) **Local Anaesthetic.** Infiltration of the buccal vestibule with localised palatal (for maxillary teeth) infiltration is sufficient for maxillary teeth. For mandibular molars in patients under

four years of age, buccal and lingual infiltration anaesthetic is sufficient for extraction. A combination of an inferior alveolar nerve block with localised buccal infiltration is required for mandibular teeth in patients over four years of age.

6) **Positioning.** The patient should be positioned lying almost flat, with the patient's head and headrest slightly raised.

7) **Elevation.** A straight elevator should be applied to the mesial and distal areas of the periodontal ligament. Using a wheel-and-axle motion, the periodontal ligament should be gently expanded until a small amount of mobility is noted in the tooth. Care must be taken to elevate between tooth and bone only, and not against adjacent teeth. The thumb and finger of the non-dominant hand should be used to support the alveolus of the tooth being extracted, to guide the application of force to the tooth socket only, and to prevent instrument slippage.

8) **Delivery.** The should be applied to the cementoenamel junction. Initially, apical pressure is used to slide the beaks as deep on to the root as possible. Slow, sustained buccolingual movements, with a predominant buccal force, should then be used to continue expansion of the socket. It is not uncommon to encounter fracture of one of the roots at this stage. Finally, the tooth should be delivered with a large buccal movement.

9) **Assessment.** The tooth root should be assessed to ensure it has been removed complete. Any remaining root fragments are likely to be loose in the socket, and can be gently removed with a straight elevator. The socket must be examined for bleeding, alveolar bone fracture, or soft tissue trauma, which should be managed as appropriate.

Bibliography

Abuabara, A., Cortez, A.L.V., Passeri, L.A. et al. (2006). Evaluation of different treatments for oroantral/oronasal communications: experience of 112 cases. *International Journal of Oral and Maxillofacial Surgery* 35 (2): 155–158.

Brockmann, W. and Badr, M. (2010). Chronic kidney disease: pharmacological considerations for the dentist. *Journal of the American Dental Association* 141 (11): 1330–1339.

Douketis, J.D. (2010). Pharmacologic properties of the new oral anticoagulants: a clinician-oriented review with a focus on perioperative management. *Current Pharmaceutical Design* 16 (31): 3436–3441.

Daly, C.G., Currie, B.J., Jeyasingham, M.S. et al. (2008). A change of heart: the new infective endocarditis prophylaxis guidelines. *Australian Dental Journal* 53 (3): 196–200.

Friedlander, A.H., Chang, T.I., Hazboun, R.C., and Garrett, N.R. (2015). High C-terminal cross-linking telopeptide levels are associated with a minimal risk of osteonecrosis of the jaws in patients taking oral bisphosphonates and having exodontia. *Journal of Oral and Maxillofacial Surgery* 73 (9): 1735–1740.

Huang, G.J. and Rue, T.C. (2006). Third-molar extraction as a risk factor for temporomandibular disorder. *Journal of the American Dental Association* 137 (11): 1547–1554.

Lababidi, E., Breik, O., Savage, J. et al. (2018). Assessing an oral surgery specific protocol for patients on direct oral anticoagulants: a retrospective controlled cohort study. *International Journal of Oral and Maxillofacial Surgery* 47 (7): 940–946.

Miller, C.S., Little, J.W., and Falace, D.A. (2001). Supplemental corticosteroids for dental patients with adrenal insufficiency: reconsideration of the problem. *Journal of the American Dental Association* 132 (11): 1570–1579.

Moore, P.A. and Hersh, E.V. (2013). Combining ibuprofen and acetaminophen for acute pain management after third-molar extractions: translating clinical research to dental practice. *Journal of the American Dental Association* 144 (8): 898–908.

Nabil, S. and Samman, N. (2011). Incidence and prevention of osteoradionecrosis after dental extraction in irradiated patients: a systematic review. *International Journal of Oral and Maxillofacial Surgery* 40 (3): 229–243.

Nabil, S. and Samman, N. (2012). Risk factors for osteoradionecrosis after head and neck radiation: a systematic review. *Oral Surgery, Oral Medicine, Oral Pathology, and Oral Radiology* 113 (1): 54–69.

Nguyen, E., Grubor, D., and Chandu, A. (2014). Risk factors for permanent injury of inferior alveolar and lingual nerves during third molar surgery. *Journal of Oral and Maxillofacial Surgery* 72 (12): 2394–2401.

Principles of Dentoalveolar Extractions, First Edition. Seth Delpachitra, Anton Sklavos and Ricky Kumar.
© 2021 John Wiley & Sons Ltd. Published 2021 by John Wiley & Sons Ltd.
Companion website: www.wiley.com/go/delpachitradentoalveolarextractions

Nunn, M.E. (2009). Essential dental treatment (EDT) in pregnant women during the second trimester is not associated with an increased risk of serious adverse pregnancy outcomes or medical events. *Journal of Evidence-Based Dental Practice* 9 (2): 91–92.

Perry, D.J., Noakes, T.J.C., and Helliwell, P.S. (2007). Guidelines for the management of patients on oral anticoagulants requiring dental surgery. *British Dental Journal* 203 (7): 389–393.

Pogrel, M.A. (2012). What are the risks of operative intervention? *Journal of Oral and Maxillofacial Surgery* 70 (9): S33–S36.

Pototski, M. and Amenábar, J.M. (2007). Dental management of patients receiving anticoagulation or antiplatelet treatment. *Journal of Oral Science* 49 (4): 253–258.

Reed, K.L., Malamed, S.F., and Fonner, A.M. (2012). Local anesthesia part 2. technical considerations. *Anesthesia Progress* 59 (3): 127–137.

Renton, T., Smeeton, N., and McGurk, M. (2001). Factors predictive of difficulty of mandibular third molar surgery. *British Dental Journal* 190 (11): 607–610.

Rood, J.P. and Shehab, B.N. (1990). The radiological prediction of inferior alveolar nerve injury during third molar surgery. *British Journal of Oral and Maxillofacial Surgery* 28 (1): 20–25.

Ruggiero, S.L., Dodson, T.B., Fantasia, J. et al. (2014). American Association of Oral and Maxillofacial Surgeons position paper on medication-related osteonecrosis of the jaw – 2014 update. *Journal of Oral and Maxillofacial Surgery* 72 (10): 1938–1956.

Seddon, H.J. (1942). A classification of nerve injuries. *British Medical Journal* 2 (4260): 237–239.

Sklavos, A., Beteramia, D., Delpachitra, S.N., and Kumar, R. (2019). The panoramic dental radiograph for emergency physicians. *Emergency Medicine Journal* 36 (9): 565–571.

Syrjänen, S.M. and Syrjänen, K.J. (1979). Influence of Alvogyl on the healing of extraction wound in man. *International Journal of Oral Surgery* 8 (1): 22–30.

Index

Principles of Dentoalveolar Extractions, First Edition. Seth Delpachitra, Anton Sklavos and Ricky Kumar.
© 2021 John Wiley & Sons Ltd. Published 2021 by John Wiley & Sons Ltd.
Companion website: www.wiley.com/go/delpachitradentoalveolarextractions